HOEKELMAN'S HANDBOOK
Primary Pediatric Care Companion

HOEKELMAN'S HANDBOOK
Primary Pediatric Care Companion

Robert A. Hoekelman, M.D.

Professor of Pediatrics
University of Rochester School of Medicine and Dentistry
Rochester, New York

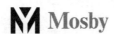 Mosby

St. Louis Baltimore Boston Carlsbad Chicago Naples New York
Philadelphia Portland London Madrid Mexico City Singapore
Sydney Tokyo Toronto Wiesbaden

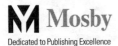

Mosby

Dedicated to Publishing Excellence

A Times Mirror Company

Publisher: Anne S. Patterson
Editor: Kathryn H. Falk
Developmental Editor: Carolyn M. Kruse
Project Manager: Patricia Tannian
Project Specialist: John Casey
Book Design Manager: Gail Morey Hudson
Cover Designer: Teresa Breckwoldt
Manufacturing Manager: Dave Graybill

Printed in the United States of America
Composition by Clarinda Company
Printing/binding by Plus Communications

Mosby–Year Book, Inc.
11830 Westline Industrial Drive
St. Louis, Missouri 63146

International Standard Book Number 0-8151-4485-7

96   97   98   99   00   /   9   8   7   6   5   4   3   2   1

Preface

During the past decade, Hoekelman's *Primary Pediatric Care,* now in its third edition, has become the primary care pediatric reference of choice for medical and nursing students, pediatric and family medicine residents, and practicing physicians and nurses. Its 5 editors and 300 authors have included within its 2000 pages all the information needed to provide care to well and sick infants, children, and adolescents.

Hoekelman's Handbook contains a collection of facts and figures from *Primary Pediatric Care,* third edition, in a pocket-sized format, ideal for quick reference or recall in ambulatory and inpatient settings. The parent text should be consulted for in-depth discussion of pertinent subjects. *Hoekelman's Handbook* is intended as an extension of *Primary Pediatric Care* rather than a substitute for it.

The facts and figures in this handbook, which represent only a small portion of those in *Primary Pediatric Care,* appear in the form of boxes, tables, figures, and algorithms directed to preventive health care; the causes, differential diagnosis, and treatment of various symptoms and diseases; and normal and abnormal values for laboratory tests and other diagnostic procedures.

Robert A. Hoekelman

PART ONE
Etiology and Classification of Common Diseases

PART TWO
Differential Diagnosis

PART THREE
Diagnostic Approach

PART FOUR
Therapeutic Modalities

PART FIVE
Medication Comparison Tables

PART SIX
Miscellaneous Information

Etiology and Classification of Common Diseases

Causes of acute abdominal pain in infancy and early childhood

Gastrointestinal causes

Meconium ileus
Hirschsprung disease
Intestinal stenosis/atresia
Infectious enteritis/gastritis
Pyloric stenosis
Malrotation
Intestinal duplication
Inguinal hernia
Intussusception
Adhesions
Appendicitis

Genitourinary causes

Testicular torsion
Urinary tract infection
Urinary obstruction
(posterior urethral valves, tumors)

Trauma

Intraluminal hematoma
Pancreatic pseudocyst

Drugs/toxins

Lead
Lactose intolerance
Salicylates
Erythromycin
Ibuprofen

Other

Sickle cell disease
Henoch-Schönlein purpura
Primary peritonitis
Pneumonia

See *Primary Pediatric Care*, ed 3, p. 852.

Causes of acute abdominal pain in late childhood and adolescence

Gastrointestinal causes

Appendicitis
Adhesions
Infectious enteritis/gastritis
Intussusception
Obstruction
Gastroesophageal reflux
Ulcer
Inguinal hernia

Genitourinary causes

Pregnancy (tubular, incomplete/
threatened abortion)
Pelvic inflammatory disease
Genital tract obstruction
(imperforate hymen with
menarche, bifid uterus)
Dysmenorrhea
Ovulation/ovarian cysts
Torsion of ovaries or testes
Undescended testicle
Urinary tract infection
Urinary calculi

Trauma

Intraluminal hematoma
Pancreatic pseudocyst

Drugs/toxins

Lead and other heavy metals
Lactose intolerance
Alcohol
Salicylates
Erythromycin
Tetracycline
Ibuprofen

Other

Sickle cell disease
Henoch-Schönlein purpura
Primary peritonitis
Pneumonia
Muscle strain/sprain
Cholecystitis
Pancreatitis
Familial Mediterranean fever
Porphyrias

See *Primary Pediatric Care*, ed 3, p. 852.

Causes of recurrent abdominal pain

Organic (see acute causes in the boxes on p. 3)

Infectious gastroenteritis (*Giardia lamblia, Salmonella, Shigella, Yersinia enterocolitica,* viral)
Peptic ulcer disease
Gastritis
Esophagitis
Hiatal hernia
Inflammatory bowel disease (Crohn disease, regional enteritis)

Dysfunctional

Constipation/chronic stool retention
Lactose intolerance
Intestinal gas with heightened awareness of intestinal motility
Dysmenorrhea
Mittelschmerz
Overeating
Irritable colon

Psychogenic

Acute reactive anxiety
School phobia
Conversion reaction
Depression
Complaint modeling
Hypochondriasis
Factitious

See *Primary Pediatric Care,* ed 3, p. 852.

Causes of airway obstruction

Congenital causes

Craniofacial dysmorphism
Hemangioma
Laryngeal cleft/web
Laryngoceles, cysts
Laryngomalacia
Macroglossia
Tracheal stenosis
Vascular ring
Vocal cord paralysis

Acquired infectious causes

Acute laryngotracheobronchitis
Diphtheria
Epiglottitis
Laryngeal papillomatosis
Membranous croup (bacterial tracheitis)
Mononucleosis
Retropharyngeal abscess
Spasmodic croup

Acquired noninfectious causes

Anaphylaxis
Angioneurotic edema
Foreign body aspiration
Supraglottic hypotonia
Thermal/chemical burn
Trauma
Vocal cord paralysis

See *Primary Pediatric Care,* ed 3, p. 1651.

Causes of primary amenorrhea

1. Familial
2. Psychosocial stress
3. Obesity or severe weight loss (similarly, thin body habitus associated with strenuous exercise programs, as seen in ballet dancers and in patients with anorexia nervosa)
4. Endocrine
   a. Hypopituitarism
   b. Congenital adrenal hyperplasia; adrenal disease
   c. Gonadal dysgenesis (Turner syndrome or Turner mosaic)
   d. Premature ovarian failure
   e. Testicular feminization syndrome
   f. Hypothyroidism
   g. Polycystic ovary disease (rare)
5. Chronic disease
6. Pregnancy
7. Anatomical anomalies
   a. Vaginal agenesis
   b. Uterine agenesis
   c. Imperforate hymen
8. Brain tumor (e.g., prolactinoma)

See *Primary Pediatric Care*, ed 3, p. 861.

Apnea of the newborn

Septicemia (e.g., meningitis or necrotizing enterocolitis)

Impaired oxygenation, hypoxemia, severe anemia, and shock or marked systemic to pulmonary circulatory shunt (e.g., patent ductus arteriosus)

Metabolic disorders (e.g., hypoglycemia, hypercalcemia, hyponatremia, hypernatremia, and hyperammonemia)

Drugs (e.g., narcotics or central nervous system depressants taken by the mother)

Central nervous system disorders (e.g., intracranial hemorrhage, seizures, or malformations of the brain)

Thermal instability (i.e., a rapid increase or decrease of temperature)

See *Primary Pediatric Care*, ed 3, p. 538.

Causes of loss of appetite in infants and children

Organic disease

Infectious (acute or chronic)

Neurological
Congenital degenerative disease
Hypothalamic lesion
Increased intracranial pressure (including a brain tumor)
Swallowing disorders (neuromuscular)

Gastrointestinal
Oral lesions (e.g., thrush or herpes simplex)
Gastroesophageal reflux
Obstruction (especially with gastric or intestinal distention)
Inflammatory bowel disease
Celiac disease
Constipation

Cardiac
Congestive heart failure (especially associated with cyanotic lesions)

Metabolic
Renal failure and/or renal tubule acidosis
Liver failure
Congenital metabolic disease
Lead poisoning

Nutritional
Marasmus
Iron deficiency
Zinc deficiency

Fever
Rheumatoid arthritis
Rheumatic fever

Drugs
Morphine
Digitalis
Antimetabolites
Methylphenidate
Amphetamines

Miscellaneous
Prolonged restriction of oral feedings, beginning in the neonatal period
Systemic lupus erythematosus
Tumor

Psychological factors

Anxiety, fear, depression, mania (limbic influence on the hypothalamus)
Avoidance of symptoms associated with meals (abdominal pain, diarrhea, bloating, urgency, dumping syndrome)
Anorexia nervosa
Excessive weight loss and food aversion in athletes, simulating anorexia nervosa

See *Primary Pediatric Care,* ed 3, p. 1052.

Causes of chest pain in children and adolescents

Cardiac disease

Anomalous coronary artery, coronary arteritis
Cardiomyopathy, myocarditis, pericarditis
Left ventricular outflow obstruction
Mitral valve prolapse
Tachyarrhythmias

Chest wall syndrome

Costochondritis, Tietze syndrome
Hypersensitive xiphoid
Muscle strain, trauma
Slipping rib syndrome
Tender breast masses

Gastrointestinal conditions

Esophageal burns, foreign bodies
Esophageal dysmotility
Esophagitis, gastritis, peptic ulcer disease

Miscellaneous

Cigarette smoking, cocaine
Fitz-Hugh-Curtis syndrome
Hemoglobinopathy with vaso-occlusive crisis
Tumors

Precordial catch syndrome

Psychogenic factors

Pulmonary conditions

Asthma, cough
Pleuritis, pleurodynia, pneumonia
Pneumomediastinum
Pneumothorax
Pulmonary embolism

See *Primary Pediatric Care,* ed 3, p. 888.

Poisons associated with coma

Alcohol
Anesthetics
Antihistamines
Barbiturates
Benzodiazepines
Butyrophenone
Bromide
Carbamates
Carbon monoxide
Clonidine
Cyanide
Hydrocarbons
Hypoglycemics (oral and injectable)
Iron
Lead
Lithium
Meprobamate
Monoamine oxidase (MAO) inhibitors
Narcotics
Organophosphates
Phenothiazines
Salicylates
Sedative-hypnotics
Strychnine
Theophylline
Tricyclic antidepressants

From Mandl KD, Lovejoy FH: *Pediatr Rev* 15:151, 1994; and Woolf AD: *Pediatr Rev* 14:411, 1993.

See *Primary Pediatric Care,* ed 3, p. 1660.

Causes of croup

Agent	Epidemiology
Most frequent	
Parainfluenza type 1	Epidemic, fall
Less frequent	
Influenza A	Epidemic, winter
Influenza B	Epidemic, winter
Respiratory syncytial virus	Epidemic, winter-spring
Mycoplasma pneumoniae	Endemic
Parainfluenza type 2	Occasionally epidemic, fall
Parainfluenza type 3	Spring to summer
Uncommon	
Adenoviruses	Endemic
Rhinoviruses	Endemic, fall, spring-summer
Reoviruses	Endemic
Coronaviruses	Epidemic, winter
Herpesvirus hominis	Endemic

See *Primary Pediatric Care,* ed 3, p. 1662.

Causes of acute diarrhea

Usually without blood in stool

Viral enteritis—reovirus (rotavirus and orbivirus), Norwalk agent, enteric adenovirus, calicivirus, and astrovirus

Enterotoxin—*Escherichia coli, Klebsiella* organisms, cholera, *Clostridium perfringens, Staphylococcus* organisms, and *Vibrio* species

Parasitic—*Giardia* and *Cryptosporidium* organisms

Extraintestinal infection—otitis media and urinary tract infection

Antibiotic-induced and *Clostridium difficile* toxin (without pseudomembranous colitis)

Commonly associated with blood in stool

Bacterial—*Shigella, Salmonella,* and *Campylobacter* organisms, *Yersinia enterocolitica,* invasive *E. coli,* gonococcus (venereal spread), enteroadherent *E. coli, Aeromonas hydrophila,* and *Plesiomonas shigelloides*

Amebic dysentery

Hemolytic-uremic syndrome

Henoch-Schönlein purpura

Pseudomembranous enterocolitis (*C. difficile* toxin)

Ulcerative or granulomatous colitis (acute presentation)

Necrotizing enterocolitis (neonates)

See *Primary Pediatric Care,* ed 3, p. 903.

Causes of chronic diarrhea

More common causes

Chronic nonspecific diarrhea (toddler's diarrhea, irritable colon of childhood)
Disaccharide intolerance
Chronic constipation with overflow diarrhea
Cystic fibrosis
Gluten-sensitive enteropathy (celiac disease)
Inflammatory bowel disease—Crohn disease and ulcerative colitis
Hirschsprung disease
Immunodeficiency states
Chronic enteric infection—*Salmonella* organisms, *Yersinia enterocolitica, Campylobacter* and *Giardia* organisms, *C. difficile* toxin, enteroadherent *E. coli,* rotavirus (in immunodeficient patients), cytomegalovirus, and HIV
Monosaccharide intolerance
Eosinophilic (allergic) gastroenteritis
Cow milk protein intolerance
Short bowel syndrome
Urinary tract infection
Factitious causes

Less common causes

Hormonal—adrenal insufficiency and hyperthyroidism
Vasoactive intestinal polypeptide–secreting tumor
Neural crest tumor and carcinoid
Intestinal lymphangiectasia
Acrodermatitis enteropathica
Intestinal stricture or blind loop
Pancreatic insufficiency with neutropenia
Trypsinogen or enterokinase deficiency
Congenital chloride-losing diarrhea
Abetalipoproteinemia
Microvillus inclusion disease
Intestinal pseudoobstruction

See *Primary Pediatric Care,* ed 3, p. 907.

Causes of disseminated intravascular coagulation

Infections

Gram negative bacteria
Neisseria meningitidis
Hemophilus influenza
Escherichia coli
Pseudomonas sp.
Enterobacter sp.
Klebsiella sp.
Serratia marcescens
Proteus sp.
Bacteroides sp.
Francisella tularensis
Salmonella typhi
Brucella abortus
Selenomonas

Gram positive bacteria
Staphylococcus aureus
Group A and B beta-hemolytic streptococcus
Streptococcus pneumoniae
Streptococcus faecalis
Streptococcus viridans
Clostridium perfringens
Clostridium welchii
Mycobacterium tuberculosis

Viruses
Varicella
Herpes zoster
Human immunodeficiency virus
Herpes simplex
Cytomegalovirus
Hepatitis B
Rubella
Rubeola
Variola
Roseola
Echovirus type 11
Arbovirus
Arenavirus

Fungi
Aspergillus
Histoplasma
Candida

Parasites
Plasmodium falciparum (malaria)

Tissue injury

Massive trauma, especially brain and crush injuries
Shock
Asphyxia/acidosis
Ischemia/infarction
Burns
Hyperthermia/hypothermia
Fat embolism
Rhabdomyolysis

See *Primary Pediatric Care,* ed 3, p. 1676.

Vascular injury

Vascular tumors including giant hemangiomata
Malignant hypertension
Respiratory distress syndrome

Immunological disorders

Collagen vascular diseases
  Systemic lupus erythematosis
  Rheumatoid arthritis
  Wegener granulomatosis
  Inflammatory bowel disease
Antiphospholipid antibodies
  Lupus anticoagulant
  Anticardiolipin antibody syndromes
Anaphylaxis
Renal allograph rejection
Hemolytic transfusion reactions

Liver disease

Advanced cirrhosis
Fulminant hepatitis
Reinfusion of ascitic fluid
Reye syndrome

Therapy-related factors

Activated prothrombin complex concentrate in-
  fusions
Massive transfusion
Warfarin administration in patients who have severe deficiencies of protein
  C or protein S
Intravenous lipid infusion

Intrauterine factors

Fetal demise of a twin
Uterine infection
Abruptio placentae
Eclampsia
Acute fatty liver of pregnancy

Malignant neoplasms

Acute leukemia, especially promyelocytic
Lymphoma
Disseminated neuroblastoma
Familial hemophagocytic reticulosis

Other causes

Massive thrombosis, especially stroke
Intravascular hemolysis
  Erythroblastosis fetalis
Snake envenomation
Severe genetic deficiencies of protein C and protein S

From Manco-Johnson MJ: *Int J Pediatr Hematol Oncol* 1:1, 1994.

Causes of dysphagia

Structural-mechanical disorders

Esophageal atresia
Esophageal web
Foreign bodies
Hiatal hernia
Paraesophageal hernia
Stricture
  Caustic
  Congenital
  Inflammatory
Tumor
Vascular ring

Motor disorders

Achalasia
Diffuse spasm
Gastrointestinal reflux
Scleroderma

Neuromuscular disorders

Acquired central nervous system
  disease
  Tumor
  Infection
  Trauma
Cerebral palsy
Dysautonomia
Muscular dystrophy
Myasthenia gravis

Inflammatory disorders

Candida albicans infection
Cytomegalovirus infection
Epidermolysis bullosa
Esophagitis
Herpes simplex infection
Ingestion of a caustic substance

See *Primary Pediatric Care*, ed 3, p. 919.

Causes of dysuria

Urinary tract infection
Urethritis
Prostatitis
Balanoposthitis
Meatal lesions
Vulvovaginitis
Kidney or bladder stones
Obstruction
Foreign bodies
Tumors
Drugs
Trauma
Sexual abuse
Hematological disorders
Perineal dermatitis (primary)
Masturbation
Psychogenic factors

See *Primary Pediatric Care*, ed 3, p. 929.

Causes of edema in children

Cardiovascular

Congestive heart failure
Acute thrombi or emboli
Vasculitis of many types

Renal

Nephrotic syndrome
Glomerulonephritis of many types
End-stage renal failure

Endocrine or metabolic

Thyroid disease
Starvation
Hereditary angioedema

Iatrogenic

Drugs (diuretics and steroids)
Water or salt overload

Hematological

Hemolytic disease of the newborn

Gastrointestinal

Hepatic cirrhosis
Protein-losing enteritis
Lymphangiectasis
Cystic fibrosis
Celiac disease
Enteritis of many types

Lymphatic abnormalities

Congenital (gonadal dysgenesis)
Acquired

See *Primary Pediatric Care,* ed 3, p. 933.

Causes of epistaxis in children

Local

1. *Trauma:* nose picking, surgery (septoplasty, turbinectomy), blunt impact (fist or instrument), foreign body, child abuse, sports, auto accident
2. *Infection:* viral, bacterial, fungal, parasitic
3. *Chronic irritation:* allergies, recurrent colds, dry environment, chronic sniffers, smoking, cocaine abuse, ciliary dysfunction, chemicals, ingestion of a caustic substance
4. *Structural abnormality:* deviated septum, vomer spur, septal perforation
5. *Drugs:* topical sprays (phenylephrine, aerosol steroids), drying agents (decongestants, antihistamines)
6. *Neoplasms:* polyps, hemangiomas, rhabdomyosarcomas, angiofibromas

Systemic

1. *Bleeding diseases:* von Willebrand, coagulation factor deficiencies, vitamin deficiencies, Osler-Weber-Rendu, idiopathic thrombocytopenia, disseminated intravascular coagulation
2. *Infections:* rheumatic fever, diphtheria, malaria, measles
3. *Neoplasms:* leukemia, lymphoma
4. *Granulomas:* Wegener, midline reticulosis, tuberculosis, sarcoidosis
5. *Medications:* antiinflammatories (aspirin, ibuprofen), anticoagulants (warfarin), steroids
6. *Cancer treatment:* chemotherapy (methotrexate), radiotherapy
7. *Hormonal influences:* menses, birth control pills, pregnancy
8. *Cardiovascular disease:* hypertension, arteriosclerosis
9. *Barometric pressure changes:* scuba diving, air flight, elevator rides
10. *Miscellaneous:* liver disease, renal dysfunction, aplastic anemia, sepsis

See *Primary Pediatric Care,* ed 3, p. 937.

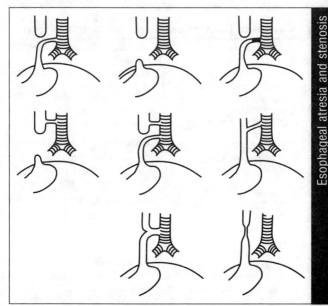

Esophageal atresia and stenosis

Types of esophageal atresia and stenosis with and without tracheoesophageal fistula.   (From Avery ME et al: *The lung and its disorders in the newborn infant,* ed 4, Philadelphia, 1981, WB Saunders.)
See *Primary Pediatric Care,* ed 3, p. 559.

Causes of failure to thrive*

Failure to thrive

Improper feeding—50%-90%

Economic—10%-40%
Education—10%-40%
Psychological—30%-40%
Intolerance—<5%

Other causes—10%-50%

Hypothyroidism
Cystic fibrosis
Subdural hematoma

Glycogen storage disease
Celiac disease
Methylmalonic acidemia
Maple syrup urine disease
Mental retardation, unspecified
Urinary tract disease
Diencephalic syndrome
Brain tumors
Chronic liver disease
Congenital heart disease
Ulcerative colitis

*Compendium from various sources. Some obvious causes are missing because the complaint is not failure to thrive but rather is related to the diagnosis.

See *Primary Pediatric Care,* ed 3, p. 951.

Causes of fever of unknown origin in children

Infectious diseases

Bacterial
  Brucellosis
  Bacterial endocarditis
  Leptospirosis
  Liver abscess
  Mastoiditis (chronic)
  Osteomyelitis
  Pelvic abscess
  Perinephric abscess
  Pyelonephritis
  Salmonellosis
  Sinusitis
  Subdiaphragmatic abscess
  Tuberculosis
  Tularemia
Viral
  Cytomegalovirus
  Hepatitis viruses
  Epstein-Barr virus
    (infectious mononucleosis)
Chlamydial
  Lymphogranuloma venereum
  Psittacosis
Rickettsial
  Q fever
  Rocky Mountain spotted fever
Fungal
  Blastomycosis (nonpulmonary)
  Histoplasmosis (disseminated)

Infectious diseases—cont'd

Parasitic
  Malaria
  Toxoplasmosis
  Visceral larva migrans
Unclassified
  Sarcoidosis

Collagen-vascular diseases

Juvenile rheumatoid arthritis
Polyarteritis nodosa
Systemic lupus erythematosus

Malignancies

Hodgkin disease
Leukemia-lymphoma
Neuroblastoma

Miscellaneous

Central diabetes insipidus
Drug fever
Ectodermal dysplasia
Factitious fever
Familial dysautonomia
Granulomatous colitis
Infantile cortical hyperostosis
Nephrogenic diabetes insipidus
Pancreatitis
Periodic fever
Serum sickness
Thyrotoxicosis
Ulcerative colitis

From Feigin RD, Cherry JD: *Textbook of pediatric infectious diseases,* ed 2, Philadelphia, 1987, WB Saunders.

See *Primary Pediatric Care,* ed 3, p. 967.

Causes of gastrointestinal hemorrhage

Infants under 1 year of age

Manifesting as upper gastrointestinal bleeding
  Swallowed maternal blood
  Gastritis, acid-peptic disease
  Stress ulceration
  Mallory-Weiss syndrome
  Vascular malformations
Manifesting as lower gastrointestinal bleeding
  Anal fissure or trauma
  Gastroenteritis
    Enteric infections
    Enterocolitis
  Intussusception
  Coagulation disorders
  Congenital malformations
    Malrotation
    Intestinal duplications, Meckel diverticulum
  Food allergies

Children over 1 year of age

Manifesting as upper gastrointestinal bleeding
  Stress ulcers
  Gastritis, acid-peptic disease
  Esophageal varices
  Esophagitis
  Mallory-Weiss syndrome
  Swallowed blood from nasopharynx
Manifesting as lower gastrointestinal bleeding
  Anal fissures
  Polyps
  Gastroenteritis, enteric infections
  Intussusception
  Inflammatory bowel disease
  Congenital malformations
    Malrotation or volvulus
    Intestinal duplication
    Meckel diverticulum
  Henoch-Schönlein purpura

See *Primary Pediatric Care,* ed 3, p. 981.

Classification of genetic-metabolic disorders*

Biochemical pathways	Subgroups	Examples
Amino acid catabolism		Phenylketonuria, homocystinuria, tyrosinemia, maple syrup urine disease, nonketotic hyperglycinemia
	Amino acid transport	Lysinuric protein intolerance, cystinuria
	Urea cycle disorders	Ornithine transcarbamylase deficiency (X-linked), citrullinemia, arginosuccinic aciduria
Organic acid metabolism		Propionic acidemia, methylmalonic acidemia, isovaleric acidemia, glutaric acidemia 1, biotinidase deficiency
Fatty acid oxidation		SCAD, MCAD, LCAD
	Fatty acid transport disorders	Carnitine transport defect, carnitine palmitoyl transferase deficiencies
Carbohydrate metabolism	Carbohydrate intolerances	Galactosemia, hereditary fructose intolerance
	Disorders of glycogen breakdown (glycogen storage disorders)	*Hepatic forms:* glucose-6-phosphatase deficiency (GSD1), debrancher enzyme deficiency (GSD 3) *Muscle form:* muscle phosphorylase deficiency (GSD 5) *Lysosomal form:* Pompe disease (GSD 2)
	Disorders of glucose catabolism (glycolysis) and synthesis (gluconeogenesis)	Pyruvate dehydrogenase deficiency, pyruvate carboxylase deficiency, fructose diphosphatase deficiency
Protein glycosylation		Carbohydrate-deficient glycoprotein syndromes

See *Primary Pediatric Care,* ed 3, p. 204.

Classification of genetic-metabolic disorders*—cont'd

Organelles	Subgroups	Examples
Peroxisomal disorders	Disorders of peroxisome assembly	Zellweger syndrome, neonatal adrenoleukodystrophy, infantile Refsum disease, rhizomelic chondrodysplasia punctata
	Single enzyme defects	X-linked adrenoleukodystrophy
Lysosomal storage disorders	Lysosomal enzyme deficiencies	*Mucopolysaccharidoses:* Hurler/Scheie (MPS 1), Hunter (MPS 2, X-linked), Sanfilippo (MPS 3) *Sphingolipidoses:* Tay-Sachs, Krabbe, metachromatic leukodystrophy, Niemann-Pick, Gaucher, Fabry (X-linked) *Glycoprotein degradation:* mannosidosis, fucosidosis
	Disorders of lysosomal enzyme transport	*Mucolipidoses:* I-cell disease (ML 2)
Mitochondrial disorders	Defects in respiratory chain complexes	Leigh syndrome (one of several causes), primary lactic acidoses, multiple acyl-CoA dehydrogenase deficiency (glutaric acidemia 2) *Mitochondrial encoded defects:* MELAS, MERRF (maternal inheritance)

*All disorders are autosomal recessive unless otherwise noted.

LCAD, Long chain acyl-CoA dehydrogenase deficiency; *MCAD,* medium chain acyl-CoA dehydrogenase deficiency; *SCAD,* short chain acyl-CoA dehydrogenase deficiency; *MPS,* mucopolysaccharidosis; *GSD,* glycogen storage disease; *ML,* mucolipidosis; *MELAS,* mitochondrial encephalomyopathy, lactic acidosis, strokelike episodes; *MERRF,* myoclonic epilepsy, ragged red fibers.

Factors associated with poor intrauterine growth

Maternal

1. Prepregnancy weight <50 kg
2. Poor nutrition; poor weight gain during pregnancy; socioeconomic factors
3. Maternal illness:
   a. Associated with uterine ischemia: hypertensive vascular disease, preeclampsia, diabetes mellitus, sickle cell anemia, autoimmune vasculitis
   b. Associated with chronic hypoxia: cyanotic congenital heart disease, high altitude
4. Drug ingestion:
   a. Drugs that affect fetal growth directly, e.g., ethanol, methadone, heroin
   b. Drugs that inhibit placental blood flow (nicotine)
5. Multiple gestation, primiparity, grand multiparity

Placental

1. Villitis associated with congenital infections (TORCH infections)
2. Ischemic villous necrosis or infarction
3. Chronic separation (abruptio placentae)
4. Diffuse fibrinosis
5. Abnormal insertion
6. Umbilical vascular thrombosis

Fetal

1. Syndromes associated with diminished birth weight; e.g., Cornelia de Lange syndrome, Potter disease, anencephaly, and dwarfism
2. Metabolic disorders (inborn errors of metabolism)
3. Chromosomal disorders: trisomies 13, 18, 21; XO
4. Congenital infections: TORCH infections, malaria, varicella

See *Primary Pediatric Care*, ed 3, p. 547.

Causes of extraglomerular hematuria

Infection (e.g., cystitis, urethritis, balinitis)
Hypercalciuria (e.g., absorptive hypercalciuria, renal tubular hypercalciuria)
Trauma (e.g., vehicular accidents, falls, child abuse)
Urinary lithiasis (e.g., hypercalciuria, cysteinuria)
Malformations (e.g., cystic kidney diseases, posterior urethral valves, ureteropelvic junction obstruction)
Hemoglobinopathy (e.g., sickle cell disease, thalassemia)
Drugs (e.g., antibiotics, cytoxan)
Bleeding diathesis (e.g., von Willebrand disease, hemophilia)
Instrumentation (e.g., suprapubic aspiration, urinary catheterization, cystoscopy, self-stimulation)
Tumors (e.g., Wilms tumor, rhabdomyosarcoma, bladder papilloma)

See *Primary Pediatric Care*, ed 3, p. 998.

Causes of hemoglobinuria and myoglobinuria

Hemoglobinuria

Hemolytic anemia (e.g., glucose-6-phosphate dehydrogenase [G6PD]
   deficiency, Coombs-positive hemolytic anemia)
Mismatched blood transfusions
Intravascular coagulation (e.g., disseminated intravascular coagulation
   [DIC], hemolytic-uremic syndrome)
Infections (e.g., sepsis, malaria)
Freshwater near-drowning
Mechanical erythrocyte damage (e.g., artificial heart valves, cardio-
   pulmonary bypass)

Myoglobinuria

Muscle injury (e.g., crush injuries, electrical burns)
Myositis
Rhabdomyolysis

See *Primary Pediatric Care,* ed 3, p. 997.

Causes of hemolytic-uremic syndrome

Infection-related

E. Coli
Shigella
Neuraminidase-producing organisms
Human immunodeficiency virus

Sporadic

Familial
Pregnancy
Transplantation
Malignant hypertension
Drugs
Tumors
Collagen-vascular disease

See *Primary Pediatric Care,* ed 3, p. 1329.

Hemoglobinuria and myoglobinuria

Hemolytic-uremic syndrome

Causes of hemoptysis in children

Infection

Bacterial
  Bronchitis
  Lung abscess
  Necrotizing pneumonia
  Tuberculosis
  Bronchiectasis
  Immune deficiency
  Cystic fibrosis
  Ciliary dyskinesia
Fungal
  Actinomycosis
  Aspergillosis
  Coccidioidomycosis
  Histoplasmosis
Parasitic
  Echinococcosis (hydatid disease)
  Paragonimiasis
  Strongyloidiasis

Foreign bodies

Congenital defects

Cardiovascular
  Congenital heart defects
  Absent pulmonary artery
  Arteriovenous malformation
  Hemangiomatous malformation
  Telangiectasia
  (Rendu-Osler-Weber syndrome)
Other
  Pulmonary sequestration
  Bronchogenic cyst
  Intrathoracic enteric cyst

Vasculitis

Periarteritis nodosa

Autoimmune disorders

Wegener granulomatosis
Pulmonary hemosiderosis
Milk allergy
Goodpasture syndrome
Collagen-vascular disease

Trauma

Compression or crush injury
Iatrogenic
  Postsurgical
  Diagnostic lung puncture
  Transbronchial biopsy
Inhalation of toxins

Neoplastic conditions

Endobronchial metastases
Primary lung tumors
  Benign (hamartoma, neurogenic tumors)
  Malignant (bronchial adenoma, bronchogenic carcinoma, pulmonary blastoma)
Endometriosis

Drug induced

Propylthiouracil

Pulmonary embolism

Hemoglobinopathy with pulmonary infarct

Factitious

See *Primary Pediatric Care*, ed 3, p. 1000.

Causes of secondary hypertension

Cause	Mechanism
Renal	Renal parenchymal disease
	Glomerulonephritis
	Chronic pyelonephritis
	Polycystic kidney
	Connective tissue disease
	Hydronephrosis
	Renal tumors
Cardiac	Coarctation of the aorta
Adrenal	Cortical
	Mineralocorticoid secreting tumors
	Adrenogenital syndrome
	Medullary
	Pheochromocytoma
Neurogenic	Increased intracranial pressure from a variety of pathological causes
Drug induced	Oral contraceptives
	Amphetamines
	Sympathomimetic amines
	Cocaine, phencyclidine (PCP), illicit drugs, licorice

See *Primary Pediatric Care,* ed 3, p. 1010.

Hypertension, secondary

Causes of hypoglycemia in childhood

Hyperinsulinism
Islet cell dysplasia (functional beta-cell secretory disorder)
Islet cell adenoma
Adenomatosis
Beckwith-Wiedemann syndrome

Hereditary defects in carbohydrate metabolism
Glycogen storage diseases
Glucose-6-phosphatase deficiency, types Ia, Ib
Amylo-1,6-glucosidase deficiency, type III
Defects of liver phosphorylase enzyme system

Enzyme deficiencies of gluconeogenesis
Fructose-1,6-diphosphatase (FDPase)
Phosphoenolpyruvate carboxykinase
Pyruvate carboxylase

Other enzyme defects
Galactose-1-phosphate uridyltransferase (galactosemia)
Fructose-1-phosphate aldolase (hereditary fructose intolerance)
Glycogen synthetase

Hereditary defects in amino acid and organic acid metabolism
Maple syrup urine disease
Propionic acidemia
Methylmalonic aciduria
Tyrosinosis
3-Hydroxy-3-methylglutaric aciduria
Glutaric aciduria, type II

Hereditary defects in fat metabolism
Systemic carnitine deficiency
Carnitine palmitoyl transferase deficiency
Long- and medium-chain acyl-CoA dehydrogenase deficiencies

See *Primary Pediatric Care,* ed 3, p. 1719.

Causes of hypoglycemia in childhood—cont'd

Hormone deficiencies

Congenital hypopituitarism or hypothalamic abnormality
Growth hormone
Cortisol
Adrenocorticotropic hormone (ACTH)
ACTH unresponsiveness
Glucagon
Thyroid hormone
Catecholamine

Ketotic hypoglycemia
Nonpancreatic tumors

Mesenchymal tumors
Epithelial tumors
Hepatoma
Adrenocortical carcinoma
Wilms tumor
Neuroblastoma

Poisoning or toxins

Salicylate
Alcohol
Propranolol
Oral hypoglycemic agents (e.g., sulfonylureas)
Insulin
Unripe ackees (hypoglycin) (Jamaican vomiting sickness)
Pentamidine

Liver disease

Hepatitis, cirrhosis
Reye syndrome

Other causes

Malnutrition
Malabsorption
Chronic diarrhea
Cyanotic congenital heart disease
Postsurgery

Modified from Cornblath MD, Schwartz R: *Disorders of carbohydrate metabolism in infancy*, ed 2, Philadelphia, 1976, WB Saunders. Originally from Kogut MD: Hypoglycemia: pathogenesis, diagnosis, and treatment. In Gluck L et al, editors: *Current problems in pediatrics*, Chicago, 1994, Mosby; and Kogut MD: Neonatal hypoglycemia: a new look. In Moss AJ, editor: *Pediatrics update: review for physicians*, New York, 1980, Elsevier.

Causes of hypothyroidism

Congenital hypothyroidism

A. Thyroid dysgenesis
  1. Thyroid aplasia
  2. Thyroid hypoplasia
  3. Ectopic thyroid gland
B. Familial abnormalities of thyroid hormone synthesis and metabolism (familial dyshormonogenesis)
C. Maternal disease
  1. Therapeutic doses of ^{131}I after the eleventh week of gestation
  2. Transplacental autoimmune thyroiditis
  3. Ingestion of goitrogens
D. Endemic goiter and cretinism
E. Hypothalamic-pituitary hypothyroidism
  1. Pituitary agenesis or aplasia
  2. Thyrotropin deficiency: isolated
  3. Hypothalamic hormone deficiency
    a. Isolated thyrotropin deficiency
    b. Multiple tropic hormone deficiencies
    c. Septooptic dysplasia
    d. Anencephaly
  4. Hypothalamic-pituitary lesions

Juvenile hypothyroidism

A. Thyroiditis, autoimmune (Hashimoto)
  1. Atrophic thyroiditis of infancy
  2. Chronic lymphocytic thyroiditis of childhood
  3. Atrophic thyroiditis of childhood and adolescence
  4. Hashimoto thyroiditis (struma lymphomatosa)
B. Congenital thyroid dysgenesis
  1. Ectopic thyroid
  2. Hypoplastic
C. Congenital defects in thyroid hormone synthesis or metabolism
D. Iatrogenic thyroid ablation
  1. Surgical
  2. Radioactive iodine (^{131}I)
E. Ingestion of goitrogens
F. Endemic goiter
G. Hypothalamic-pituitary disease

See *Primary Pediatric Care,* ed 3, p. 1358.

Immunodeficiency syndromes

Humoral-mediated immunodeficiency
Antibody deficiency syndromes

Transient hypogammaglobulinemia of infancy
X-linked infantile hypogammaglobulinemia
Common variable immunodeficiency or acquired hypogammaglobu-
    linemia
Isolated IgA deficiency
Isolated IgM deficiency
Antibody deficiency with normal immunoglobulins
Miscellaneous dysgammaglobulinemias

Leukocyte deficiency syndromes

Decreased number of leukocytes
    Marrow toxicity
    Immune injury to marrow
    Myelothisic suppression of marrow
    Familial hypoplasia
Defective leukocyte function
    Chronic granulomatous disease
    Chédiak-Higashi disease
    Lazy leukocyte syndrome

Complement deficiency syndromes

Isolated C3 deficiency
Isolated C5 deficiency
C2 and C4 deficiencies

Cell-mediated immunodeficiency

Congenital thymic hypoplasia (DiGeorge syndrome)
Chronic mucocutaneous candidiasis

Mixed B and T cell immunodeficiency

HIV infection
Severe combined immunodeficiency
Wiskott-Aldrich syndrome
Immunodeficiency with ataxia-telangiectasia
Immunodeficiency with thymoma
Immunodeficiency with short-limbed dwarfism
Cellular immune deficiency with abnormal immunoglobulin synthesis
    (Nezelof syndrome)

See *Primary Pediatric Care*, ed 3, p. 1093.

Etiology of lymphadenopathy

Differential diagnosis	Newborn	Infant	Child	Adolescent
Infections				
Bacterial				
Pyogenic	Group B streptococci	Streptococci/staphylococci, and other gram positive and gram negative organisms →		
			Cat-scratch fever →	
			Typhoid fever →	
			Tularemia →	
Spirochetal	Syphilis →			Syphilis
				Anaerobes
				Vincent angina
Granulomatous		Mycobacteria →		
		Atypical mycobacteria →		
Viral				→HHV6 syndrome
			Rubella →	
			Rubeola →	
			Varicella →	
		Adenovirus →		
		Enterovirus →		
			Epstein-Barr virus (EBV) →	
			Cytomegalovirus (CMV) →	
			Herpes simplex virus (HSV) (stomatitis, pharyngitis, or skin infection) →	
		Human immunodeficiency virus (HIV) →		
Protozoan	Toxoplasmosis →			
Fungal		Histoplasmosis →		
		Other fungi (rare cases) →		

See *Primary Pediatric Care,* ed 3, p. 1054.

Rickettsial   Rocky Mountain spotted fever ———— Lymphogranuloma →
Chlamydial
Parasitic   Toxocara ———— →
    Myiasis ———— →

Neoplastic

Endogenous   Leukemia ———— →
    Lymphoma ———— →
    Histiocytosis ———— →
    Hodgkin disease ———— →

Exogenous   Neuroblastoma ———— →
(Metastatic)   Wilms tumor ———— →
    Ewing sarcoma ———— →
    Rhabdomyosarcoma ———— →

Immunological

    Juvenile rheumatoid arthritis (JRA) ———— →
    Systemic lupus erythematosus (SLE) ———— →
    Serum sickness ———— →
    Sarcoidosis ———— →

Other

(Reactive)   Kawasaki disease ———— →
    Hemoglobinopathies ———— →
    Hemophilia ———— →
    Phenytoin ———— →
    Addison disease ———— →
    Hyperthyroidism ———— →

Chronic granulomatous disease (CGD) ———— →
Agammaglobulinemia ———— →

Malformation syndromes associated with congenital hemangiomas

Condition	Nature of hemangioma	Other features
Sturge-Weber syndrome	Large, flat hemangioma over face; usually involves ophthalmic branch of trigeminal nerve; usually unilateral	Seizures Glaucoma Mental deficiency
Kasabach-Merritt syndrome	Usually large cavernous hemangiomas, although small ones have been reported	Thrombocytopenia from platelet sequestration
Klippel-Trenaunay-Weber syndrome	Large, flat hemangioma on an extremity	Hemangioma overlies area of soft tissue and bone overgrowth Macrocephaly
Diffuse neonatal hemangiomatosis	Multiple hemangiomas that can involve skin and internal organs	High-output cardiac failure; poor prognosis

See *Primary Pediatric Care*, ed 3, p. 528.

Infectious agents associated with illnesses in which petechial or purpuric exanthems, or both, occur

Infectious agent	Illness
Varicella-zoster virus	Hemorrhagic chickenpox
Cytomegalovirus	Congenital cytomegalovirus infection
Variola virus	Hemorrhagic smallpox
Coxsackieviruses A4, A9	Fever
Coxsackieviruses B2 to B4	Exanthem and enanthem
Echoviruses 4, 7, 9	
Colorado tick fever virus	Colorado tick fever
Rotavirus	Gastroenteritis
Alphaviruses	Chikungunya fever, o'nyong-nyong fever, Ross River fever, Sinbis fever
Rubella virus	Rubella (German measles)
	Congenital rubella
Respiratory syncytial virus	Bronchiolitis
Measles virus	Hemorrhagic (black) measles
	Atypical measles
Lassa virus	Lassa fever
Marburg virus	Hemorrhagic fever
Rickettsia typhi	Murine typhus
Rickettsia prowazekii	Epidemic typhus
Rickettsia rickettsii and other tickborne rickettsiae	Rocky Mountain spotted fever
Ehrlichia canis	Ehrlichiosis
Mycoplasma pneumoniae	Atypical pneumonia
Streptococcus pyogenes	Scarlet fever; septicemia
Streptococcus pneumoniae	Pneumococcal septicemia
Enterococcal and viridans group streptococci	Endocarditis
Neisseria gonorrhoeae	Gonococcemia
Neisseria meningitidis	Meningococcemia
Moraxella catarrhalis	Sinusitis, otitis media, sepsis
Haemophilus influenzae	*H. influenzae* septicemia
Pseudomonas aeruginosa	Ecthyma gangrenosum
Streptobacillus moniliformis	Rat-bite fever
Yersinia pestis	Septicemic plague (Black Death)
Bartonella henselae	Cat-scratch fever
Treponema pallidum	Congenital syphilis
Borrelia spp.	Relapsing fever
Toxoplasma gondii	Congenital toxoplasmosis
Trichinella spiralis	Trichinosis

Modified from Cherry JD: Cutaneous manifestations of systemic infections. In Feigen RD, Cherry JD, editors: *Textbook of pediatric infectious diseases*, Philadelphia, 1992, WB Saunders.

See *Primary Pediatric Care,* ed 3, p. 1731.

Causes of recurrent pneumonia

Aspiration

Gastroesophageal reflux
Tracheoesophageal fistula
Altered consciousness (i.e., seizures)
Foreign body
Abnormal swallowing reflex

Structural causes

Pulmonary sequestration
Tracheal or bronchial stenosis/web
Extrinsic compression of the airway
   Vascular ring
   Lymph nodes

Immunological deficiency

Acquired: AIDS, chemotherapy, malnutrition
Congenital: humoral, phagocytic

Metabolic causes

Cystic fibrosis
Alpha-1-antitrypsin deficiency

Altered mucociliary clearance

Immotile cilia syndrome

Other

Asthma
Hypersensitivity pneumonitis

See *Primary Pediatric Care*, ed 3, p. 1522.

Causes of delayed puberty

I. Constitutional delay
II. Deficiency of GnRH secretion by the hypothalamus
   A. Genetic
      1. Isolated deficiency
      2. Kallmann syndrome
      3. Laurence-Moon-Bardet-Biedl syndrome
      4. Prader-Willi syndrome
   B. Acquired
      1. Infection
      2. Neoplasm
      3. Infiltrative disease
      4. Trauma

Causes of delayed puberty—cont'd

III. Deficiency of gonadotropin secretion by the pituitary
   A. Genetic
      1. Panhypopituitarism
      2. Isolated deficiency
      3. Fertile eunuch (normal FSH, low LH)
   B. Acquired
      1. Infection
      2. Neoplasm
      3. Trauma
IV. Gonadal disorders
   A. Genetic
      1. Turner syndrome (45, X or structural X abnormalities or mosaicism)
      2. Klinefelter syndrome (47, XXY abnormality)
      3. Noonan syndrome
      4. Syndromes of complete androgen insensitivity (no sexual hair)
      5. Del Castillo syndrome (Sertoli cells only)
      6. Pure gonadal dysgenesis
      7. Myotonic dystrophy
   B. Acquired
      1. Infections
         a. Gonorrhea (male)
         b. Virus (usually mumps)
         c. Tuberculosis (male)
      2. Radiotherapy or chemotherapy
      3. Mechanical causes
         a. Torsion
         b. Surgery
         c. "Vanishing testes"
      4. Autoimmune
V. Adrenal and gonadal steroid enzyme deficiencies
VI. Chronic systemic diseases
   A. Congenital heart disease
   B. Chronic pulmonary disease
   C. Inflammatory bowel disease
   D. Chronic renal failure and renal tubular acidosis
   E. Hypothyroidism
   F. Poorly controlled diabetes mellitus
   G. Sickle cell anemia
   H. Collagen-vascular disease
   I. Anorexia nervosa

See *Primary Pediatric Care,* ed 3, p. 1105.

Causes of heterosexual precocious puberty

I. Female
   A. Congenital adrenal hyperplasia
   B. Androgen-secreting tumors
      1. Adrenal
      2. Ovarian
      3. Teratoma
   C. Exogenous androgens
II. Male
   A. Estrogen-producing tumors
      1. Adrenal
      2. Teratoma
      3. Hepatoma
      4. Testicular
   B. Exogenous estrogens
   C. Increased peripheral conversion of androgens to estrogens

See *Primary Pediatric Care,* ed 3, p. 1107.

Causes of isosexual precocious puberty

I. Central (with pituitary gonadotropin secretion)
   A. Idiopathic
   B. Central nervous system abnormalities
      1. Congenital anomalies (hydrocephalus)
      2. Tumors (hypothalamic, pineal, other)
      3. Hamartoma
      4. Postinflammatory condition
      5. Trauma
      6. Syndromes
         a. Neurofibromatosis
         b. Tuberous sclerosis
   C. Hypothyroidism (severe)
II. Pseudoprecocious puberty
   A. Exogenous sex steroids
   B. Gonadal tumors or cysts
   C. Adrenal hyperplasia or tumor
   D. Ectopic gonadotropin-secreting tumors (chorioepithelioma, hepatoblastoma, teratoma)
   E. Familial Leydig cell hyperplasia
   F. McCune-Albright syndrome

See *Primary Pediatric Care,* ed 3, p. 1106.

Causes of obstructive pulmonary disease

Newborns

Choanal atresia or stenosis
Dermoid cyst
Encephalocele
Hemangioma
Vocal cord paralysis
Pierre Robin syndrome
Ankyloglossia (Tongue tie)
Pertussis

Infants

Foreign body
Vascular ring
Tracheal web
Bronchiolitis
Asthma
Cystic fibrosis
Bronchomalacia
Pyogenic thyroid
Accessory thyroid

Children and adolescents

Foreign body
Asthma
Adenopathy
  Lymphoma
  Systemic lupus erythematosus
  Tuberculosis
  Sarcoidosis
Croup
Epiglottitis
Retropharyngeal abscess
Enlarged tonsils or adenoids
Cystic fibrosis
Anaphylaxis
Laryngeal tumor
Vocal cord tumor
Tracheal tumors
Vocal cord polyp
Laryngeal trauma
Supraglottitis
Diphtheria
Bacterial tracheitis
Ingestion of caustic substance
Crack cocaine

Pulmonary disease, obstructive

See *Primary Pediatric Care,* ed 3, p. 924.

Causes of restrictive pulmonary disease

Newborns

Hyaline membrane disease
Hypoplastic lungs
Eventration of the diaphragm
Meconium aspiration
Pneumonia (group B streptococci
  or gram negative organisms)
Diaphragmatic paralysis
Osteogenesis imperfecta
CNS depression
  Hypoxia
  Congenital
  Maternal drugs
Congenital myasthenia gravis
Aspiration
Pulmonary edema
  Septicemia
  Congenital heart disease

Infants

Pneumonia
  Bacterial
  Viral
  Aspiration
Bronchopulmonary dysplasia
Wilson-Mikity syndrome
Hamman-Rich syndrome
Pulmonary edema
Infantile botulism
Congenital lobar emphysema

Children and adolescents

Skeletal
  Kyphoscoliosis
  Ankylosing spondylitis
  Pectus excavatum
  Crush chest injury

Parenchymal
  Pneumonia
  Hypersensitivity pneumonitis
  Systemic lupus erythematosus
  Scleroderma
  Fibrosis
  Toxin inhalation
  Granulomatous disease
  Drugs (e.g., antineoplastic
    agents and narcotics)
  Carcinoma
  Fat embolus
  Pneumothorax
Smoke inhalation
Pulmonary infarction
Pulmonary edema
  Congestive heart failure
  Sepsis
  Intracranial disease
  Croup
  Epiglottitis
Neuromuscular
  Cord transection
  Myasthenia gravis
  Muscular dystrophy
  Multiple sclerosis
  Guillain-Barré syndrome
  Pickwickian syndrome
  Toxins
Pleural effusion
  Pneumonia
  Hypoproteinemia
  Renal failure
  Tumor
  Pulmonary infarction

See *Primary Pediatric Care*, ed 3, p. 924.

Causes of respiratory distress in the newborn

Pulmonary causes
Common

Hyaline membrane disease
Transient tachypnea of the newborn (TTN)
Meconium aspiration
Primary pulmonary hypertension

Occasional

Pulmonary hemorrhage
Pneumonia
Pneumothorax
Pulmonary dysmaturity

Rare

Airway obstruction
   Choanal atresia
Space-occupying lesion
   Diaphragmatic hernia
   Cysts
   Tumors

Nonpulmonary causes
Cerebral

Hemorrhage
Edema

Metabolic

Acidosis
Hypoglycemia
Hypothermia

Hematological

Hypovolemia
   Acute blood loss
   Twin-to-twin transfusion
Hyperviscosity

See *Primary Pediatric Care,* ed 3, p. 550.

Causes of Reye syndrome

Infections

Meningitis
Varicella
Hepatitis
Encephalitis

Inborn metabolic defects

Systemic carnitine deficiency
Hyperammonemia syndromes
Organic acid disorders

Anoxic encephalopathy

Toxins

Salicylates
Methyl bromide
Hypoglycin
Isopropyl alcohol
Aflatoxin
Lead
Valporic acid

See *Primary Pediatric Care,* ed 3, p. 1545.

Causes of scrotal swelling

Acute, painful scrotal swelling

Torsion of spermatic cord
Torsion of appendix, testis, epididymis
Acute epididymitis, orchitis
Mumps orchitis
Henoch-Schönlein purpura
Trauma
Insect bite
Thrombosis of spermatic vein
Fat necrosis
Hernia
Folliculitis
Dermatitis

Acute, painless scrotal swelling

Tumor
Idiopathic scrotal edema
Hydrocele
Henoch-Schönlein purpura
Hernia

Chronic scrotal swelling

Hydrocele
Hernia
Varicocele
Spermatocele
Sebaceous cyst
Tumor

See *Primary Pediatric Care,* ed 3, p. 1100.

Classification of seizures and epilepsy syndromes

Primary generalized
Seizure types

Absence
Myoclonic
Atonic/astatic
Tonic-clonic

Epilepsy syndromes

Infantile spasms (West syndrome)
Lennox-Gastaut syndrome
Childhood absence epilepsy
Juvenile myoclonic epilepsy

Partial
Seizure types

Simple partial
Complex partial
Partial seizures with secondary generalization

Epilepsy syndromes

Benign partial epilepsy of childhood
Epilepsia partialis continua

Unclassified

Neonatal seizures
Febrile seizures
Pseudoseizures

*Data from Commission on Classification and Terminology of the International League Against Epilepsy: *Epilepsia* 26:268, 1985.

See *Primary Pediatric Care*, ed 3, p. 1564.

Advanced trauma life support classification of shock

Class I

15% or less loss of acute blood volume
Blood pressure normal
Age-related pulse increased 10% to 20%
No change in capillary refill

Class II

20% to 25% loss of blood volume
Tachycardia >150 beats/min
Tachypnea 35 to 40 breaths/min
Capillary refill prolonged >3 sec
Systolic blood pressure decreased
Pulse pressure decreased
Orthostatic hypotension
Urine output >1 ml/kg/hr

Class III

30% to 35% blood volume loss
All of the above signs
Urine output <1 ml/kg/hr
Lethargic, clammy skin, and vomiting

Class IV

40% to 50% blood volume loss
Nonpalpable pulses
Obtunded

See *Primary Pediatric Care,* ed 3, p. 1763.

Classification of shock

Hypovolemic

Dehydration
Gastrointestinal losses
Blood loss
Excess urine output
  Diabetes mellitus
  Diabetes insipidus
High-output renal failure
"Third space" fluid losses
  Peritonitis
  Burns
  Hypoalbuminemia
Mannitol administration
Diuretic agent administration

Distributive

Septic shock
Hypoadrenal states
Anaphylaxis
Drug overdose

Cardiogenic

Pump or inotropic
  Myocarditis
  Myocardiopathy
  Decreased contractility acquired in sepsis syndromes
  Hypoplastic left heart syndrome
  Arrhythmia
Obstructive
  Coarctation of the aorta
  Tamponade caused by excessive pericardial blood, fluid, or air

See *Primary Pediatric Care,* ed 3, p. 1762.

Disorders associated with paranasal sinusitis

1. Anatomical
   a. Nasal malformations
   b. Nasal trauma
   c. Tumors and polyps
   d. Cleft palate
   e. Foreign bodies
   f. Dental infection
   g. Cyanotic congenital heart disease
2. Physiological—barotrauma
3. Abnormalities of local defense mechanisms
   a. Allergy
   b. Cystic fibrosis
   c. Immotile-cilia syndrome and Kartagener syndrome
4. Abnormalities of systemic defense mechanisms—
   immunodeficiency, primary or secondary

From Shurin PA: *Ann Otol Rhinol Laryngol* 90(suppl 84):72, 1981.

See *Primary Pediatric Care,* ed 3, p. 1594.

Some causes of splenomegaly

Infections

Viral: Epstein-Barr, cytomegalovirus, human immunodeficiency virus
Bacterial: acute bacterial infections, subacute bacterial endocarditis, congenital syphilis, tuberculosis
Protozoal: malaria, toxoplasmosis
Fungal: candidiasis, histoplasmosis, coccidioidomycosis

Hematological disorders

Hemolytic anemias—congenital and acquired
    Red cell membrane defects: hereditary spherocytosis, hereditary elliptocytosis
    Red cell hemoglobin defects: sickle cell disease and related syndromes, thalassemia
    Red cell enzyme defects: pyruvate kinase deficiency and others
    Autoimmune hemolytic anemia
Extramedullary hematopoiesis
    Thalassemia major, osteopetrosis, myelofibrosis

Infiltrative disorders

Leukemias
Lymphomas
Lipidoses
Mucopolysaccharidosis
Histiocytosis X

Congestive splenomegaly

Chronic congestive heart failure
Portal hypertension secondary to hepatic cirrhosis

Inflammatory diseases

Systemic lupus erythematosus (SLE)
Rheumatoid arthritis (Still disease)
Serum sickness
Sarcoidosis
Immune thrombocytopenias and neutropenias

Primary splenic disorders

Cysts
Hemangiomas and lymphangiomas
Subcapsular hemorrhage

See *Primary Pediatric Care,* ed 3, p. 1108.

Classification of predispositions to chronic stool retention

Altered anatomy or physiology

Congenital
  Aganglionic megacolon
  Anal stenosis or atresia
Acquired
  Postoperative lesion
  Fissure
  Celiac disease
Metabolic
  Hypothyroidism
  Hypocalcemia
  Multiple endocrine neoplasia
  Drug effects (especially
    codeinelike medications
    and phenothiazines)
Neurogenic (myelodysplasia)

Dysfunctions

Developmental
  Associated with cognitive
    handicap
  Attentional disorders or
    hyperactivity
Situational
  Associated with difficult
    training
  School bathroom induced
  Negative defecation-related
    experience (e.g., gastroen-
    teritis)
Psychogenic—associated with
  significant psychopathology
Constitutional
  Primary colonic inertia
  Genetic predisposition

See *Primary Pediatric Care,* ed 3, p. 892.

Causes of acute stridor in pediatric patients

Infectious

Laryngotracheobronchitis
  (croup)
Epiglottitis
Bacterial tracheitis
Retropharyngeal abscess
Peritonsillar abscess
Severe adenotonsillitis (infec-
  tious mononucleosis)
Ludwig angina
Diphtheria
Membranous croup

Immune-mediated

Anaphylaxis
Angioneurotic edema

Trauma

Foreign body (in larynx, trachea,
  or esophagus)
Laryngeal fracture
Cricoarytenoid dislocation
Hematoma
Caustic ingestion
Thermal/inhalation injury

Metabolic

Hypocalcemia (vocal cord
  tetany)
Biotinidase deficiency

See *Primary Pediatric Care,* ed 3, p. 1123.

Causes of chronic/frequently recurrent stridor in pediatric patients

Nasal cavity

Bilateral choanal atresia
Anterior encephalocele
Polyps
Neoplasms
Dermoid cysts

Oropharynx/nasopharynx

Craniofacial dysmorphia (micrognathia and glossoptosis; e.g., Pierre Robin and Treacher Collins syndromes)
Macroglossia (e.g., Beckwith syndrome, congenital hypothyroidism, glycogen storage disease, lingual thyroid)
Hyperplasia of the tonsils and adenoids
Thyroglossal duct cyst
Cystic hygroma

Supraglottic area

Laryngomalacia
Cysts of vallecular, epiglottis, arytenoids
Laryngeal web
Papillomatosis

Glottic and subglottic area

Vocal cord paralysis
Psychogenic stridor (paradoxical vocal cord motion)
Glottic and subglottic webs
Subglottic stenosis (congenital and acquired)
Subglottic hemangioma

Trachea

Tracheal stenosis
Tracheomalacia
Vascular rings and slings
Enlarged thyroid
Spasmodic croup

Esophagus

Esophageal atresia
Tracheal-esophageal fistula
Laryngotracheal-esophageal cleft
Gastroesophageal reflux
Achalasia

Mediastinal masses

Bronchogenic cysts
Ectopic thymus
Neoplasm
Enlarged lymph nodes

See *Primary Pediatric Care,* ed 3, p. 1123.

Differential Diagnosis

Differential diagnosis of acute lower abdominal pain in the adolescent female by organ system

Urinary

Cystitis
Pyelonephritis
Urethritis
Other

Gastrointestinal

Appendicitis
Constipation
Diverticulitis
Gastroenteritis
Inflammatory bowel disease
Irritable bowel syndrome
Other

Reproductive

Acute PID
Cervicitis
Dysmenorrhea (primary/secondary)
Ectopic pregnancy
Endometriosis
Endometritis
Mittelschmerz
Ovarian cyst (torsion/rupture)
Pregnancy (intrauterine, ectopic)
Ruptured follicle
Septic abortion
Threatened abortion
Torsion of adnexa
Tuboovarian abscess

From Shafer M, Sweet RL: *Pediatr Clin North Am* 36:513, 1989.

Abdominal pain, acute lower, in adolescent female

See *Primary Pediatric Care,* ed 3, p. 1590.

Primary acid-base abnormalities and their expected compensatory changes

Disorder	Primary abnormality	Associated abnormalities	Expected compensatory changes if simple disorder exists
Metabolic acidosis	Elevation in hydrogen ion concentration ($\downarrow$ pH)	$\downarrow$ Bicarbonate concentration and total CO_2; negative base excess	PCO_2 will fall by 1.5 times the fall in bicarbonate concentration (maximum change is 10 mm Hg)
Respiratory acidosis	Elevation in PCO_2	$\uparrow$ Hydrogen ion concentration and total CO_2; $\downarrow$ pH	Bicarbonate concentration rises by 3.5-4 mEq/L for each 10 mm Hg rise in PCO_2 (cannot be above 30 mEq/L if the problem is short term, 45 if long term)
Metabolic alkalosis	Decreased hydrogen ion concentration ($\uparrow$ pH)	$\uparrow$ Bicarbonate concentration and total CO_2; positive base excess	PCO_2 rises by 0.5-1 mm Hg for every 1 mEq rise in bicarbonate concentration (to a maximum of 55 mm Hg)
Respiratory alkalosis	Decreased PCO_2	$\downarrow$ Hydrogen ion concentration and total CO_2; $\uparrow$ pH	Bicarbonate concentration falls by 2.5-5 mEq/L for each 10 mm Hg fall in PCO_2 (lower limit is 18 mEq/L if short term, 12-15 mEq/L if long term)

See *Primary Pediatric Care*, ed 3, p. 337.

Differential diagnosis of childhood acute leukemia

Nonmalignant conditions

Juvenile rheumatoid arthritis
Systemic lupus erythematosus
Infectious mononucleosis
Idiopathic thrombocytopenic purpura
Pertussis, parapertussis
Aplastic anemia
Acute benign infectious lymphocytosis
Leukemoid reaction (more common in ANLL)
Bacterial sepsis with or without coagulopathy (more common in ANLL)
Osteomyelitis

Malignancies

Neuroblastoma
Lymphoma (especially if mediastinal mass, massive adenopathy, and organomegaly are present)
Retinoblastoma
Rhabdomyosarcoma
Ewing sarcoma
Chronic myelogenous leukemia

Unusual presentations

Hypereosinophilic syndrome
Cord compression or cauda equina syndrome
Eosinophilic granuloma
Parenchymal brain lesion

See *Primary Pediatric Care*, ed 3, p. 1402.

Differential diagnosis of appendicitis

Common conditions
  Gastroenteritis
  Constipation
Medical problems
  Urinary tract infection
  Diabetic ketoacidosis
  Sickle cell crisis
  Right lower lobe pneumonia
  Primary peritonitis
  Inflammatory bowel disease
Gynecological problems
  Pelvic inflammatory disease
  Ovarian torsion
  Ruptured ectopic pregnancy
  Dysmenorrhea
  Mittelschmerz
Unusual conditions
  Henoch-Schönlein purpura
  Hemolytic-uremic syndrome
  Rocky Mountain spotted fever
Surgical emergencies
  Meckel diverticulitis
  Intestinal adhesions
  Intussusception
  Necrotizing enterocolitis

See *Primary Pediatric Care*, ed 3, p. 1188.

Differential diagnosis of juvenile arthritis

Rheumatic disease of childhood

Acute rheumatic fever
Systemic lupus erythematosus
Juvenile ankylosing spondylitis
Polymyositis and dermatomyositis
Vasculitis
Scleroderma
Psoriatic arthritis
Mixed connective tissue disease
  and overlap syndromes
Kawasaki disease
Behçet syndrome
Familial Mediterranean fever
Reiter syndrome
Reflex sympathetic dystrophy
Fibromyalgia (fibrositis)

Infectious diseases

Bacterial arthritis
Viral or postviral arthritis
Fungal arthritis
Osteomyelitis
Reactive arthritis

Neoplastic diseases

Leukemia
Lymphoma
Neuroblastoma
Primary bone tumors

Noninflammatory disorders

Trauma
Avascular necrosis syndromes
Osteochondroses
Slipped capital femoral epiphysis
Diskitis
Patellofemoral dysfunction (chon-
  dromalacia patellae)
Toxic synovitis of the hip
Overuse syndromes

Genetic or congenital syndromes

Hematological disorders

Sickle cell disease
Hemophilia

Inflammatory bowel disease

Miscellaneous

Growing pains
Psychogenic arthralgias (conver-
  sion reactions)
Hypermobility syndrome
Villonodular synovitis
Foreign body arthritis

See *Primary Pediatric Care,* ed 3, p. 1384.

Differential diagnosis of coma in adolescents

Supratentorial causes

Arteriovenous malformation
Hemorrhage
Hydrocephalus
  Malfunction of ventricular shunt
Trauma
Tumor

Subtentorial causes

Arteriovenous malformation
Basilar artery migraine

Metabolic causes

Asphyxiation
  Autoerotic
Drug overdose
Encephalitis
Hepatic failure
Hypertension
  Encephalopathy
Hyperthermia
  Heat stroke
Hypothermia
Hypothyroidism
Hypoglycemia
Hypoxia
Meningitis
Occupational exposure to toxins
Poisoning
Pulmonary disease
  Hypoxia
  Hypercarbia
Renal failure
Seizures/postictal state
Sepsis
Shock
Suicide attempt
Vasculitis
  Lupus erythematosus
  Epstein-Barr virus

See *Primary Pediatric Care*, ed 3, p. 1656.

Differential diagnosis of coma in children

Supratentorial causes

Arteriovenous malformation
Hydrocephalus
  Malfunction of ventricular shunt
Trauma
Tumor

Subtentorial causes

Arteriovenous malformation
Basilar migraine
Cerebellar abscess
Trauma

Metabolic causes

Acidosis
Altered temperature regulation
Encephalitis
Hepatic failure
Hypertension
  Encephalopathy
Hypoglycemia
Hyponatremia
Hypoxia
Meningitis
Poisoning
Pulmonary disease
  Hypoxia
  Hypercarbia
Renal failure
Seizures/postictal state
Sepsis
Shock
Suicide attempt

See *Primary Pediatric Care*, ed 3, p. 1656.

Differential diagnosis of coma, general causes*

Supratentorial causes

Closed head trauma
  Concussion
  Hemorrhage
Hemorrhage/infarction secondary
  to vascular disease
Neoplasms
  Herniation, obstruction of ce-
  rebrospinal fluid, invasion
  of activating structures
Subdural empyema

Subtentorial causes

Arteriovenous malformation
Basilar migraine
Cerebellar abscess
Cerebrovascular disease
Rupture of vertebrobasilar artery
  aneurysm

Trauma
  Posterior fossa subdural hematoma

Metabolic causes

Acid-base disorders
Altered temperature regulation
Central nervous system (CNS)
  infection or inflammation
Dysfunction of non-CNS organs
  Endocrine
  Nonendocrine
  Sepsis
Electrolyte disorders
Failure to provide substrate
  Hypoglycemia
  Hypoxia
  Ischemia
Poisoning

*These causes apply to all pediatric age groups.

See *Primary Pediatric Care,* ed 3, p. 1656.

Differential diagnosis of coma in infants

Supratentorial causes

Hydrocephalus
Intraventricular hemorrhage
Subdural empyema
Trauma
  Closed head trauma
  Shaken baby syndrome
  Subdural hematoma

Subtentorial causes

Arteriovenous malformation
Subdural hemorrhage

Metabolic causes

Asphyxiation (child abuse)
Encephalitis
Epilepsy/postictal state

Hypoglycemia
Hyponatremia
Hypothermia
Hypoxia
Inborn errors of metabolism
  Carbohydrate metabolism
  Amino acid metabolism
Intentional poisoning (child abuse)
Intussusception
Meningitis
Sepsis
Shock

See *Primary Pediatric Care,* ed 3, p. 1656.

Comparison of aganglionic megacolon and chronic dysfunctional stool retention

Characteristic	Aganglionic megacolon	Stool retention
Prevalence	1 in 25,000 births	1.5% of 7-yr-old boys
Sex ratio	90% males	86% males
Retention as newborn	Almost always	Rare
Problems with bowel training	Rare	Common
Late onset of symptoms (after 2 yr)	Rare	Common
Toilet avoidance	Rare	Common
Incontinence	Rare	Common
Stool size	Often thin "ribbons"	Often large caliber
Frequency of defecation	Greatly diminished	Variable
Abdominal pain	Rare, except in obstruction	Common, especially in cases of recent onset
General appearance	Often chronically ill	Usually healthy
Failure to thrive	Common	Rare
Obstruction	Common	Rare
Abdominal distention	Common	Variable
Stool in ampulla	Often diminished	Often increased
Plain roentgenograms	Narrow rectum	Often dilated, distended rectum
Rectal manometry (internal sphincter)	Contraction or no response	Relaxation
Barium enema	Localized constriction with proximal dilation	Often diffuse megacolon

See *Primary Pediatric Care,* ed 3, p. 891.

Causes of emesis by usual age of earliest onset

Infancy
Gastrointestinal tract

Congenital
  Regurgitation—chalasia, gastroesophageal reflux
  Atresia—stenosis (tracheoesophageal fistula, prepyloric diaphragm, intestinal atresia)
  Duplication
  Volvulus (errors in rotation and fixation, Meckel diverticulum)
  Congenital bands
  Hirschsprung disease
  Meconium ileus (cystic fibrosis), meconium plug

See *Primary Pediatric Care,* ed 3, p. 1152.   *Continued*

Causes of emesis by usual age of earliest onset—cont'd

Acquired

Acute infectious gastroenteritis, food poisoning (staphylococcal, clostridial)

Pyloric stenosis

Gastritis, duodenitis

Intussusception

Incarcerated hernia—inguinal, internal secondary to old adhesions

Cow milk protein intolerance, food allergy, eosinophilic gastroenteritis

Disaccharidase deficiency

Celiac disease—presents after introduction of gluten in diet, inherited risk

Adynamic ileus—the mediator for many nongastrointestinal causes

Neonatal necrotizing enterocolitis

Chronic granulomatous disease with gastric outlet obstruction

Nongastrointestinal tract

Infectious—otitis, urinary tract infection, pneumonia, upper respiratory tract infection, sepsis, meningitis

Metabolic—aminoaciduria and organic aciduria, galactosemia, fructosemia, adrenogenital syndrome, renal tubular acidosis, diabetic ketoacidosis, Reye syndrome

Central nervous system—trauma, tumor, infection, diencephalic syndrome, rumination, autonomic responses (pain, shock)

Medications—anticholinergics, aspirin, alcohol, idiosyncratic reaction (e.g., codeine)

Childhood (additional causes)
Gastrointestinal tract

Peptic ulcer—vomiting is a common presentation in children younger than 6 years old

Trauma—duodenal hematoma, traumatic pancreatitis, perforated bowel

Pancreatitis—mumps, trauma, cystic fibrosis, hyperparathyroidism, hyperlipidemia, organic acidemias

Crohn disease

Idiopathic intestinal pseudoobstruction

Superior mesenteric artery syndrome[7]

Nongastrointestinal tract

Central nervous system—cyclic vomiting, migraine, anorexia nervosa, bulimia

Characteristic signs of epiglottitis compared with viral croup and bacterial tracheitis

	Epiglottitis	Viral croup	Bacterial tracheitis
Peak age	3-7 yr	3 mo-3 yr	Any age (mostly ≤12 yr)
History	Previously well	Preceding upper respiratory tract infection common; may have had croup previously	Preceding upper respiratory tract infection common; sometimes viral croup; occasionally previous trauma or manipulation of trachea and upper respiratory tract
Onset	Acute (hours)	Less acute (days)	Acute (hours)
Appearance	Toxic; drooling, dysphagia; sitting forward, mouth open	Less toxic; no drooling	Toxic; respiratory distress and stridor; drooling and sitting forward not characteristic
Cough	Unusual	Very characteristic, spasmodic, "seal's bark"	May be absent or may be present from preceding viral upper respiratory tract infection
Temperature	High (usually 39° C)	Lower (usually <39° C, sometimes none)	High (usually >39° C)
Pharynx	"Beefy" erythema	Normal or slight erythema	Normal or minimal inflammation
White blood cell count and differential	High; left shift	Normal or slight increase; normal or slight left shift	High; left shift
Roentgenogram of neck	"Thumb" sign on lateral view (edematous epiglottis)	Subglottic narrowing on posteroanterior view	Normal epiglottis; subglottic narrowing with membranous tracheal exudate occasionally visible on lateral view

See *Primary Pediatric Care*, ed 3, p. 1703.

Differentiating common childhood exanthems

Disease	Character of rash	Prodrome	Pathognomonic signs	Helpful signs
Enterovirus infection	Maculopapular; generalized to most of body; discrete	May have 3-4 days of mild fever before rash, or rash may appear with constitutional signs	Herpangina, hand-foot-mouth syndrome	Aseptic meningitis, pharyngitis, petechiae with some coxsackievirus strains; occurs in summer and early fall
Exanthem subitum (roseola)	Maculopapular and discrete; begins on trunk and spreads to face and limbs	3-4 days of high fever and irritability with no other signs	None	Dramatic drop in fever simultaneous with onset of rash
Erythema infectiosum (fifth disease)	Red and flushed cheeks with circumoral pallor; maculopapular rash on extremities (lacelike)	None	Slapped-cheek appearance in otherwise healthy child	Possible recurrence of eruption with irritation of skin by heat, cold, or pressure
Rubella (German measles)	Pink, maculopapular, discrete; begins on face and spreads to trunk and extremities	Commonly none; adolescents may have 1-3 days of low-grade fever and malaise	None	Tender postauricular and suboccipital lymph nodes; possibly arthralgia in adolescents
Mumps	Maculopapular, discrete, concentrated on trunk; may have urticaria	1-2 days of fever, headache, and malaise	None	Diffuse swelling of parotid glands, with pain and tenderness; aseptic meningitis; orchitis or pancreatitis; erythema of the Stensen duct
Infectious mononucleosis	Macular or maculopapular and discrete; when associated with ampicillin administration, is confluent (morbilliform) and more intense	2-4 days of fever, pharyngitis, malaise	None	Exudative pharyngitis, lymphadenopathy, splenomegaly, atypical lymphocytes on peripheral smear

See *Primary Pediatric Care,* ed 3, p. 1262.

Disease	Rash	Prodrome/Timing	Enanthem	Associated findings
Mycoplasma pneumonia	Maculopapular on trunk and extremities in 10% of cases; common spectrum of urticaria, erythema multiforme, and vesicular/bullous lesions	3-5 days of progressive fever, headache, malaise, and cough	None	Pneumonia, cold agglutinins may be elevated
Rubeola (measles)	Red to brown macular rash that spreads from face and neck to trunk and extremities; confluent (morbilliform), particularly on face; fades after 6-7 days with temporary staining of skin	3-4 days of high fever, conjunctivitis, cough, and coryza	Koplik spots	Always an associated conjunctivitis and cough
Atypical measles	Rash may be maculopapular, purpuric, petechial, or vesicular; prominent at wrists and ankles	2-3 days of fever, headache, and cough	None	History of killed measles vaccine, myalgia, pneumonia
Scarlet fever	Erythematous papular eruption sometimes associated with generalized erythema; concentrated on trunk and proximal extremities; feels like fine sandpaper	Occurs within 1-4 days of onset of focal infection	None	Focal infections such as pharyngitis, vaginitis, cellulitis, erythema of palms and soles; strawberry tongue; desquamation in recovery phase
Kawasaki disease	Rash ranges from maculopapular to scarlatina form to urticaria; marked erythema of palms and soles	1-3 days of fever and irritability	None	Conjunctivitis, tender lymphadenopathy, strawberry tongue, meatitis, diarrhea, meningitis, prolonged fever, late desquamation, arthritis in recovery phase

Differential diagnosis of a patient who is chronically fatigued

Malignancy
Autoimmune disease
Localized infection (e.g., sinusitis, occult abscess)
Chronic or subacute infection (e.g., Lyme disease, endocarditis, tuberculosis)
HIV infection
Fungal disease (e.g., Candidiasis, histoplasmosis, coccidioidomycosis, blastomycosis)
Parasitic disease (e.g., toxoplasmosis, giardiasis)

Chronic inflammatory disease (e.g., sarcoidosis, Wegener granulomatosis)
Endocrine disease (e.g., hypothyroidism, Addison disease, diabetes)
Neuromuscular disease (e.g., myasthenia gravis, multiple sclerosis)
Drug dependency
Side effects of chronic medications or other toxic agents (e.g., chemical solvent, heavy metal, pesticide)
Psychiatric disorder

See *Primary Pediatric Care,* ed 3, p. 1245.

Disorders commonly associated with prolonged fatigue

Severe anemia
Hypothyroidism
Chronic upper respiratory tract infections
  Otitis media and sinusitis
  Tonsillitis
Mycoplasma and other viral pneumonias
Infectious mononucleosis
Hepatitis
Chronic asthma
Chronic allergies
Rheumatoid arthritis

Rheumatic fever
Lupus erythematosus
Diabetes mellitus
Disseminated malignancy
Inflammatory bowel disease
AIDS
Immunological disorders
Drug abuse, including alcoholism
Cyanotic heart disease
Chronic pulmonary disease
Chronic renal failure
Depression
Severe obesity

See *Primary Pediatric Care,* ed 3, p. 953.

Pediatric gastrointestinal obstruction, clinical findings

Etiology	Vomiting	Pain	Stool pattern	Findings Distention	Bowel sounds	Tenderness	Masses
Esophageal atresia	Nonbilious (saliva)	No	Normal meconium	No	Absent to normal	No	No
Gastric obstruction	Nonbilious (curdled formula)	Severe with gastric volvulus; none with antral web	Normal meconium	Epigastric	Absent to normal	Severe with volvulus	No
Hypertrophic pyloric stenosis	Nonbilious, projectile	No	Constipation (dehydration)	Epigastric	Hyperactive (epigastric)	No	Yes ("olive")
Duodenal obstruction	Bilious	Minimal	Small meconium stool	Epigastric	Absent to normal	No	No
Volvulus	Bilious	Severe	Hematochezia	Epigastric to generalized	Hyperactive	Yes (severe)	No
Jejunoileal atresia	Bilious	No	Small, hard, light-colored meconium stool	Generalized	Variable	No	No
Intussusception	Bilious	Yes (crampy)	Currant jelly stool	Generalized	Hyperactive	Yes	Yes ("sausage shaped")
Meconium ileus	Bilious	No	Obstipation	Generalized	Variable	No	Yes ("doughy beads")
Meconium plug	Bilious	No	Obstipation	Generalized	Variable	No	No
Congenital aganglionosis	Bilious	No	Obstipation, constipation, and intermittent diarrhea	Generalized	Hyperactive	No	Palpable stool
Obstipation of prematurity	Bilious	No	Obstipation	Generalized	Hyperactive	No	No
Incarcerated inguinal hernia	Bilious	Yes	Diarrhea or constipation	Generalized	Hyperactive	Yes	Inguinal or scrotal
Imperforate anus	Bilious	No	Obstipation	Generalized	Hyperactive	No	No

See *Primary Pediatric Care*, ed 3, p. 1311.

Roentgenographic findings in gastrointestinal obstruction

	Findings				
Etiology	Dilated area	Air or fluid levels	Calcium deposits	Noncalcium opacities	Further studies that may be indicated
Esophageal atresia	Esophagus and stomach	Yes (gastric)	No	No	Esophageal air instillation
Gastric obstruction	Stomach	Yes	No	No	Gastric barium instillation*
Hypertrophic pyloric stenosis	Stomach	Yes	No	No	Ultrasonography
Duodenal obstruction	Stomach, duodenum (double bubble)	Yes	No	No	None
Volvulus	Variable	Variable	No	No	Upper GI series or barium enema
Jejunoileal atresia	Stomach and small intestine	Yes	Yes (with prenatal perforation)	No	Barium enema to rule out nonrotation
Intussusception	Stomach and small intestine	Variable	No	Yes (soft tissue densities)	Ultrasonography and/or barium enema†
Meconium ileus	Stomach and small intestine	No	Yes (meconium peritonitis)	Yes (ground-glass appearance)	Water-soluble contrast enema†
Meconium plug	Stomach to colon	Yes	No	No	Barium enema‡
Congenital aganglionosis	Stomach to colon	Yes	No	No	Barium enema
Obstipation of prematurity (short left colon syndrome)	Stomach to colon	Yes	No	No	Barium enema‡
Incarcerated inguinal hernia	Stomach and small intestine	Yes	No	No	None
Imperforate anus	Stomach to colon	Yes	No	No	Complete evaluation of genitourinary tract

*Should be performed cautiously to avoid aspiration.
†Should be performed cautiously to avoid bowel perforation.
‡May be therapeutic and diagnostic.

See *Primary Pediatric Care,* ed 3, p. 1313.

Common genetic disorders

Disorder	Manifestation	Frequency/10,000 births
Chromosomal		
Trisomy 21	Congenital heart disease, Brushfield spots, short hands, clinodactyly, simian crease, hypotonia, dysmorphic facies	16
Trisomy 18	Congenital heart disease, small for gestational age (SGA), clenched fist, rocker-bottom foot, dysmorphic facies	3
Trisomy 13	Congenital heart disease, SGA, polydactyly, holoprosencephaly, dysmorphic facies	2
XO	Congenital peripheral edema, webbed neck, short stature, primary amenorrhea	3
XXY	Behavior problems, small testes, infertility, clinodactyly	5
Autosomal recessive		
Sickle cell disease	Anemia, infection	20 (African American)
Beta-Thalassemia	Anemia	20 (Mediterranean)
Cystic fibrosis	Failure to thrive, malabsorption, cough, recurrent pneumonia	5 (Caucasian)
Autosomal dominant		
Familial hypercholesterolemia	Family history of early coronary artery disease	20
Neurofibromatosis	Café-au-lait spots	3
X-linked recessive		
Fragile X	Mental retardation, large testes, dysmorphic facies	5
Duchenne muscular dystrophy	Muscle weakness, pseudohypertrophy of calf	1

See *Primary Pediatric Care*, ed 3, p. 449.

Common causes of heart failure: differential diagnosis

Pulmonary overcirculation

Ventricular septal defect
Patent ductus arteriosus
Transposition of the great arteries
Truncus arteriosus

Vascular obstruction

Coarctation of the aorta
Aortic valve stenosis
Pulmonary valve stenosis
Pericardial tamponade

Decreased pump function

Hypoplastic ventricle
Cardiomyopathy, carditis
Prolonged tachycardia
Sepsis

Fluid overload

Renal failure
Anemia
Overhydration

See *Primary Pediatric Care,* ed 3, p. 1713.

Acute viral hepatitis

Characteristics	Virus A	Virus B	Virus C
Age distribution	Children and young adults	All age groups	All age groups
Route of infection	Predominantly fecal-oral	Parenteral-oral	Parenteral-oral
Incubation period (days)	15-40	50-180	20-90
Onset	Acute	Insidious	Insidious
Duration of clinical illness	Weeks	Weeks to months	Weeks to months
Virus present			
Feces	Late incubation, acute	May be present	Absent
Blood	Late incubation, acute	Late incubation, acute, may persist for months to years	Present chronically
Clinical features			
Fever	High, common early	Moderate, less common	Moderate, less common
Nausea and vomiting	Common	Less common	Less common
Anorexia	Severe	Mild to moderate	Mild to moderate
Arthralgia or arthritis	Rare	Common	?
Rash or urticaria	Rare	Common	?
Laboratory findings			
Aminotransferase elevation	1-3 wk	Months	Fluctuates for months
Bilirubin elevation	Weeks	May be months	Unusual
HB_sAg	Absent	Present	Absent
Severity	Usually mild	Often severe	Usually mild
Progression to chronic hepatitis	Rare	More common	High chronicity rate
Immunity	Homologous, lifelong (?)	Homologous, lifelong (?)	?
Prevention	Immune serum globulin	Hyperimmune globulin; vaccine	Screen donor blood

Modified from Krugman S, Katz SL: *Infectious diseases of children*, ed 8, St Louis, 1985, Mosby; and deBelle RC, Lester R: *Pediatr Clin North Am* 22:948, 1975.

See *Primary Pediatric Care*, ed 3, p. 1339.

Causes of increased ICP in children

Head trauma

Cerebral edema
Intracerebral hemorrhage
Extracerebral hemorrhage (subdural, epidural)

Vascular causes

Arterial/venous infarctions
Intracerebral hemorrhage
Dural sinus thrombosis
Subarachnoid hemorrhage
Vascular anomalies (vein of Galen malformation, AVMs)

Neoplastic causes

Primary brain tumors
Metastatic (intracerebral, meningeal infiltration)

Hydrocephalus

Congenital or acquired
Communicating or noncommunicating

Pseudotumor cerebrii (benign intracranial hypertension)

CNS infections

Meningitis (bacterial, fungal, mycobacterial)
Encephalitis (focal or diffuse)
Abscess

Metabolic causes

Inborn errors of metabolism (hyperammonemia)
Hepatic encephalopathy
Diabetic ketoacidosis
Renal failure
Reye syndrome
Hypoxic-ischemic encephalopathy
Fluid-electrolyte abnormalities (hyponatremia, hypernatremia)

Structural causes

Craniosynostosis

Status epilepticus

Adapted from Pickard JD, Czosnyka M: *J Neurol Neurosurg Psychiatry* 56:845, 1993.

See *Primary Pediatric Care,* ed 3, p. 1726.

Differential diagnosis of jaundice in the neonate and young infant

Unconjugated hyperbilirubinemia* (noncholestatic jaundice)

Overproduction of bilirubin

Sepsis
Rh/ABO incompatibility
Hematoma (birth trauma)
Drugs (e.g., vitamin K)
Polycythemia
Maternal-fetal or twin-to-twin transfusion
Delayed clamping of umbilical cord
Erythrocyte defects (e.g., congenital spherocytosis)
Hemoglobinopathies
Physiological jaundice

Impaired transport of bilirubin

Hypoxia, acidosis
Drugs (e.g., sulfonamides, aminosalicylic acid [ASA])
Serum free fatty acids
  Breast milk
  Fat emulsions
Hypoalbuminemia of prematurity

Impaired hepatic uptake of bilirubin

Decreased sinusoidal perfusion (e.g., diminished venous flow after birth)
Gilbert syndrome
Physiological jaundice

Impaired conjugation of bilirubin

Breast milk jaundice
Drugs (e.g., chloramphenicol)
Hypoglycemia
Hypothyroidism
High intestinal obstruction
Glucuronyl transferase deficiency (types I and II)
Physiologic jaundice

Enterohepatic circulation of bilirubin

Delayed passage of meconium
  Low intestinal obstruction
  Cystic fibrosis
Diminished intestinal motility
Physiological jaundice
Negligible intestinal bacterial flora
Presence of intestinal beta-glucuronidase

Continued.

See *Primary Pediatric Care,* ed 3, p. 1034.

Differential diagnosis of jaundice in the neonate and young infant—cont'd

Conjugated hyperbilirubinemia* (cholestatic jaundice)

Acquired cholestatic jaundice

Sepsis
Other infections
  Bacterial
  Congenital (TORCH)
  Viral (e.g., hepatitis A, B, or C; HIV)
  Parasitic (e.g., toxoplasmosis)
Chemical liver injury (e.g., drugs)
Total parenteral nutrition (TPN)

Idiopathic cholestatic jaundice

Hepatocellular cholestatic jaundice
  Neonatal hepatitis
Ductal cholestatic jaundice
  Biliary atresia
  Biliary hypoplasia
  Paucity of intrahepatic bile ducts
  Choledochal cyst

Inherited cholestatic jaundice

Familial cholestatic syndromes (e.g., benign recurrent cholestasis)
Metabolic cholestasis
  Galactosemia
  Hereditary fructose intolerance
  Hereditary tyrosinemia
  Cystic fibrosis
  Alpha-1-antitrypsin deficiency
  Glycogen storage disease
  Inborn errors of bile acid metabolism
Other storage diseases
  Niemann-Pick disease
  Gaucher disease
"Noncholestatic" syndromes
  Dubin-Johnson syndrome
  Rotor syndrome

*When this is the predominant form of bilirubin, the following diagnoses should be considered.

Differential diagnosis of jaundice in the older infant and child

Unconjugated hyperbilirubinemia* (noncholestatic jaundice)

Overproduction of bilirubin
Hemoglobinopathies (e.g., sickle cell disease)
Erythrocyte defects (e.g., congenital spherocytosis)

Impaired uptake of bilirubin
Gilbert syndrome

Impaired conjugation of bilirubin
Glucuronyl transferase deficiency (types I and II)

Conjugated hyperbilirubinemia* (cholestatic jaundice)

Acquired cholestatic jaundice
Sepsis
Other infections
  Bacterial (e.g., syphilis, leptospirosis)
  Viral (e.g., hepatitis A, B, C, D, and E; HIV, Epstein-Barr virus)
  Parasitic (e.g., toxoplasmosis)
Chemical liver injury
Drugs (e.g., valproic acid, erythromycin, sulfonamides, isoniazid, methyl-dopa)
Total parenteral nutrition (TPN)

Idiopathic cholestatic jaundice
Autoimmune hepatitis
Sclerosing cholangitis

Inherited cholestatic jaundice
Wilson disease
Cystic fibrosis
Alpha-1-antitrypsin deficiency

*When this is the predominant form of bilirubin, the following diagnoses should be considered.

See *Primary Pediatric Care*, ed 3, p. 1034.

Clinical features of Kawasaki disease and other mucocutaneous diseases

	Kawasaki disease	Stevens-Johnson syndrome	Streptococcal scarlet fever
Age (yr)	Usually <5	Usually 3-30	Usually 5-10
Fever	Prolonged	Prolonged	Variable
Eyes	Hyperemia of ocular conjunctivae; uveitis	Catarrhal conjunctivitis; chemosis; iritis; uveitis; panophthalmitis	No change
Lips	Red, dry, fissured	Erosions; crusted, fissured, bleeding	No change
Oral cavity	Diffuse erythema; "strawberry tongue"	Erythema; bullae, ulcers, pseudomembrane formation	Pharyngitis; palatal petechiae; "strawberry tongue"
Peripheral extremities	Erythema of palms and soles; indurative tive edema; periungual, palmar, and plantar desquamation	No change	Periungual desquamation
Exanthem	Erythematous, polymorphous	Erythematous, polymorphous; iris lesions, vesicles, bullae, crusts	Finely papular erythroderma; Pastia lines; circumoral pallor
Cervical lymph nodes	Nonpurulent swelling; unilateral (frequent)	Nonpurulent swelling (occasional)	Nonpurulent or purulent swelling (frequent)
Other	Meatitis; diarrhea; arthralgia and arthritis; vomiting; aseptic meningitis; rhinorrhea (uncommon); ECG changes	Malaise; cough, rhinorrhea, pneumonitis; vomiting; arthralgia; recurrent episodes	Malaise; vomiting; headache

See *Primary Pediatric Care*, ed 3, p. 1392.

Clinical features of Kawasaki disease and other mucocutaneous diseases—cont'd

	Staphylococcal scarlet fever	Staphylococcal toxic shock syndrome	Leptospirosis
Age (yr)	Usually 2-8	Usually adolescent	Usually >2
Fever	Variable	Usually <10 days	Variable
Eyes	Hyperemia of ocular conjunctivae	Hyperemia of ocular conjunctivae	Hyperemia of ocular conjunctivae; uveitis
Lips	No change	Red	No change
Oral cavity	Pharyngitis	Erythema; pharyngitis	Pharyngitis
Peripheral extremities	No change	Swelling of hands and feet; dry gangrene	Gangrene of hands and feet (rare)
Exanthem	Finely papular erythroderma; Pastia lines	Erythroderma	Erythematous, maculopapular, petechial, or purpuric
Cervical lymph nodes	Nonpurulent or purulent swelling (occasional)	No change	Nonpurulent swelling (infrequent)
Other		Headache; confusion; hypotension; icteric hepatitis; diarrhea; coagulopathy; renal injury	Headache; myalgia; abdominal pain; icteric hepatitis; meningitis

Odor as a clue to infection

Odor	Infection
Foul, putrid breath or sputum	Lung abscess, empyema (especially anaerobic), bronchiectasis, fetid bronchitis
Severe halitosis	Trench mouth, tonsillitis, gingivitis
Ammoniacal urine	Urinary tract infection with urea-splitting bacteria
Musty or grapelike, especially in a patient with burns or wounds	*Pseudomonas* skin infection
Fetid sweat	Intranasal foreign body
Rancid stool	Shigellosis
Fishy vaginal discharge	Bacterial vaginosis
Foul vaginal discharge	Vaginal foreign body
Pus that smells like feces or overripe cheese	Proteolytic bacteria
Foul cerumen	*Pseudomonas* infection
Putrid smell from skin	Scurvy
Sweetish odor from mouth	Diphtheria
Butcher shop	Yellow fever
Beer odor in peritoneal dialysate	*Candida* infection
Mousy	*Proteus* infection
Rotten apples	*Clostridium* gas gangrene
Stale beer	Scrofula
Fresh-baked brown bread	Typhoid fever
Alcohol smell to cerebrospinal fluid	*Cryptococcus* meningitis
Malodorous newborn	Amnionitis

Modified from Hayden GF: *Postgrad Med J* 67:110, 1980; Smith M, Smith LG, Levinson B: *Lancet* 2:1452, 1982; Schiffman SS: *N Engl J Med* 308:1337, 1983.

See *Primary Pediatric Care,* ed 3, p. 1066.

Inhalations, poisonings, and ingestions associated with recognizable odors

Odor	Site	Substance implicated
Fruity, like acetone or decomposing apples	Breath	Lacquer, chloroform, salicylates
Fruity, alcohol	Breath	Alcohol, phenol
Fruity, pearlike, acrid	Breath	Chloral hydrate, paraldehyde
Wintergreen	Breath	Methyl salicylate
Severe bad breath	Breath	Amphetamines
Bitter almond	Breath	Cyanide (chokecherry, apricot pits), jetberry bush
Burned rope	Breath	Marijuana
Camphor	Breath	Naphthalene (mothballs)
Coal gas	Breath	Coal gas (associated with odorless but toxic carbon monoxide)
Disinfectant	Breath	Phenol, creosote
Garlic	Breath	Phosphorus, arsenic, tellurium, parathion, malathion
Metallic	Breath	Iodine
	Stool	Arsenic
	Vomitus	Arsenic, phosphorus
Shoe polish	Breath	Nitrobenzene
Stale tobacco	Breath	Nicotine
Hydrocarbon	Breath, vomitus	Hydrocarbons
Violets	Urine, vomitus	Turpentine
Medicinal	Urine	Penicillins
Sulfides or amines	Skin	War gases

Modified from Hayden GF: *Postgrad Med* 67:110, 1980; McMillan JA, Nieburg PI, Oski FA: Diseases and poisonings associated with unusual breath odor. In *The whole pediatrician catalog*, Philadelphia, 1977, WB Saunders; Goldfrank L, Kirstein R: *Hosp Phys* 3:12, 1976; Smith M, Smith LG, Levinson B: *Lancet* 2:1452, 1982.

See *Primary Pediatric Care*, ed 3, p. 1066.

Some other diseases associated with specific odors

Disease	Odor
Diabetic ketoacidosis, starvation	Ketones are present in the breath and smell fruity, like acetone or decomposing apples
Uremia	Fishy smell to urine caused by dimethylamine and trimethylamine
	Ammoniacal smell to the breath caused by ammonia
Acute tubular necrosis	Urine smells like stale water
Hepatic failure	Breath smells like musty fish, raw liver, feces, or newly mown clover; caused by mercaptans and/or dimethyl sulfide
Intestinal obstruction, esophageal diverticulum	Breath smells feculent, foul
Schizophrenia	Sweat smells unpleasant, pungent, heavy; caused by trans-3-methyl-2-hexanoic acid
Skin diseases with protein breakdown	Skin smells foul, unpleasant
Intestinal obstruction, peritonitis	Vomitus smells like feces
Malabsorption	Stool smells foul
Portacaval shunt, portal vein thrombosis	Breath smells sweet

Modified from Hayden GF: *Postgrad Med J* 67:110, 1980; McMillan JA, Nieburg PI, Oski FA: Diseases and poisonings associated with unusual breath odor. In *The whole pediatrician catalog*, Philadelphia, 1977, WB Saunders; Smith M, Smith LG, Levinson B: *Lancet* 2:1452, 1982.

See *Primary Pediatric Care*, ed 3, p. 1066.

Extremity pain in childhood: a differential diagnosis

Allergy/collagen-vascular origin
Dermatomyositis
Familial Mediterranean fever
Inflammatory bowel disease
Juvenile rheumatoid arthritis
Mixed connective tissue disease
Polyarteritis nodosa
Rheumatic fever
Henoch-Schönlein purpura
Scleroderma
Serum sickness
Systemic lupus erythematosus

Congenital origin
Caffey disease
Hemophilia
Mucolipidosis
Mucopolysaccharidosis
Popliteal artery entrapment syndrome
Sickle cell anemia/thalassemia

Endocrine origin
Hypercortisolism
Hyperparathyroidism
Hypothyroidism

Idiopathic origin
Fibromyalgia
Growing pains
Sarcoidosis

Infectious origin
Bacterial
Arthralgia/myalgia associated with
  streptococcal infection
Diskitis
Gonorrhea
Osteomyelitis
Pyogenic myositis
Septic arthritis
Enteric disease
Histoplasmosis

Immunization reaction
Kawasaki disease
Lyme disease
Meningococcal disease
Syphilis: periostitis
Trichinosis
Tuberculosis
Viral
  Myalgia/arthralgia
  Myositis
  Toxic synovitis

Metabolic origin
Carnitine palmitoyl transferase deficiency
Fabry disease
McArdle syndrome
Phosphofructokinase deficiency

Neoplastic origin
Histiocytosis X
Leukemia

Continued.

See *Primary Pediatric Care,* ed 3, p. 941.

Extremity pain in childhood: a differential diagnosis—cont'd

Neoplastic origin—cont'd

Lymphoma
Neuroblastoma
Tumors of bone
  Chondrosarcoma
  Ewing sarcoma
  Osteoblastoma (benign)
  Osteogenic sarcoma
  Osteoid osteoma (benign)
Tumors of soft tissue
  Fibrosarcoma
  Rhabdomyosarcoma
  Synovial cell sarcoma
Tumors of the spinal cord

Nutritional origin

Gout
Hypercholesterolemia
Hypervitaminosis A

Osteoporosis
Rickets (vitamin D)
Scurvy (vitamin C)

Orthopedic origin

Chondromalacia patellae
Freiberg disease
Inflexible flat feet/tarsal coalition
Köhler disease
Legg-Calvé-Perthes disease
Osgood-Schlatter disease
Osteochondritis dissecans
Osteogenesis imperfecta
Pathological fracture
Sever disease
Slipped capital femoral epiphysis

Psychosocial origin

Behavior disorders
Psychogenic pain

Reflex neurovascular dystrophy
School phobia

Trauma/overuse

Carpal tunnel syndrome
Cervical disk syndrome
Compartment syndrome
Fracture
Hypermobility syndrome
Myohematoma
Myositis ossificans
Physical abuse
Shin splint
Sprain
Stress fracture
Subluxed radial head
Thoracic outlet syndrome

Modified from Bowyer SL, Hollister JR: *Pediatr Clin North Am* 31:5, 1984.

Differential diagnosis of polyuria in childhood

I. Neurogenic vasopressin deficiency
  A. Idiopathic
    1. Familial
    2. Sporadic
  B. Organic
    1. Posttraumatic
    2. Vascular event
    3. After infection
    4. CNS tumor
    5. Systemic infiltrative diseases (histiocytosis, syphilis, tuberculosis, sarcoidosis)
    6. Guillain-Barré syndrome
    7. Congenital intracranial defect
    8. Autoimmune disorders

II. Excessive fluid intake
  A. Primary polydipsia
  B. Water intoxication

III. Renal vasopressin insensitivity
  A. Congenital
    1. Hereditary nephrogenic diabetes insipidus
    2. Other renal tubular defects (cystinosis, distal renal tubular acidosis, Bartter syndrome)
    3. Structural defect
  B. Acquired
    1. Postinfectious
    2. Postobstructive
    3. Drug induced
    4. Associated with systemic disease (sickle cell disease, sarcoidosis, amyloidosis)
    5. Metabolic (hypercalcemia, hypokalemia)

IV. Osmotic diuresis
  A. Diet induced
  B. Drug induced
  C. Insulin-dependent diabetes mellitus
  D. Non-insulin-dependent diabetes mellitus
  E. Renal glycosuria

See *Primary Pediatric Care,* ed 3, p. 1074.

Differential diagnosis of proptosis in children

Capillary hemangioma
Craniosynostosis
Dermoid cyst
Glaucoma (secondary buphthalmos)
Histiocytosis-X
Hyperthyroidism
Idiopathic inflammatory pseudotumor
Leukemia
Lymphangioma
Meningoencephalocele
Neuroblastoma
Neurofibroma
Orbital cellulitis
Optic nerve glioma
Rhabdomyosarcoma
Trauma

See *Primary Pediatric Care,* ed 3, p. 1535.

Laboratory studies and characteristics of skin lesions in children with a rash

Diagnosis or differential diagnosis	Laboratory studies	Comments
Macule		
Erythematous		
Sunburn, phototoxic reaction		Look for patterns and sharp edges, e.g., clothing lines after exposure to sun
Rubeola		Koplik spots, preauricular lymph nodes
Drug reaction*	Leukocytosis with eosinophilia	History of drug ingestion
Toxic shock syndrome	Blood, throat, urine, stool, vaginal cultures for *Staphylococcus aureus* or *Streptococcus pyogenes*	Shock, tampon use
Infectious mononucleosis*	Heterophil antibody; atypical lymphs on smear	Generalized adenopathy, splenomegaly; ampicillin use
Kawasaki disease*	Thrombocytosis 3-5 wk after onset	Conjunctival injection, cervical adenopathy
Staphylococcal scalded skin syndrome	*S. aureus* cultured from focus	Tender erythema, positive Nikolsky sign, bullae
Toxic epidermal necrolysis	*S. aureus* cultures negative	Search for new drug use
Erythema multiforme, Stevens-Johnson syndrome	Skin biopsy may aid diagnosis	Central papule or vesicle, iris lesions; may be bullous
Viral exanthem*	Leukocytosis with lymphocytosis	Postauricular lymphadenopathy; monarticular arthritis
Rubella	Fourfold rise in antibody titer	Eruption appears with resolution of fever; periorbital edema
Roseola infantum (exanthem subitum)	Leukopenia may be present	Reticulated pattern may appear for months with stress; arthritis
Erythema infectiosum	Lymphocytosis, eosinophilia	Acute rheumatic fever with active carditis; fleeting
Erythema marginatum*		Arthritis; lesions may be papular
Juvenile rheumatoid arthritis*	Rheumatoid factor may be positive	Muscle weakness; periungual telangiectasia; heliotrope eyelid edema; Gottron papule
Dermatomyositis*	Electromyography, creatinine phosphokinase, aldolase	

See *Primary Pediatric Care*, ed 3, p. 1083.

Condition	Diagnostic Test	Comment
Lyme disease	Most nonspecific; may look for antibodies to *Borrelia burgdorferi* (see Chapter 228 on Lyme disease)	Erythema chronicum migrans appearing as enlarging rings after tick bite
Hypopigmented		
Tinea versicolor*	Potassium hydroxide (KOH) smear—short, branched hyphae and spores	Chronic; prevalent if immunosuppressed
Pityriasis alba	Wood light—hypopigmented	
Vitiligo in evolution	Wood light—depigmented if vitiliginous; T_4, TSH to rule out thyroid disorder	Observe for scleroderma, melanoma
Hyperpigmented		
Tinea versicolor*	See above	See above
Transient neonatal pustular melanosis	Pustule gram stain—sterile with polymorphonuclear neutrophils (PMNs)	Pustules; superficial desquamation
Nonblanching (petechiae, purpura)		
Atypical measles	Complete blood count (CBC), liver enzymes, viral titers	History of killed measles vaccine; pneumonitis; acral petechiae, purpura, vesiculobullous lesions
Viral exanthem, TORCH infection, drug, hepatitis*		Drug history
Rocky Mountain spotted fever*	Fluorescent antibody screen; OX-19, OX-2; skin biopsy of fluorescent stain	History of tick bite
Leukemia, coagulation defect, ITP	CBC, PT, PTT, platelet count, bone marrow aspirate and biopsy	
Battered child syndrome*		History incongruous with pattern and/or degree of lesions

Continued.

Laboratory studies and characteristics of skin lesions in children with a rash—cont'd

Diagnosis or differential diagnosis	Laboratory studies	Comments
Papules, nodules		
Erythematous		
Miliaria rubra (heat rash)		Prominent in occluded areas
Seborrheic dermatitis		Intertriginous with yellow greasy scale, cradle cap
Atopic dermatitis	IgE level	Family or personal history of allergies, asthma, eczema; flexural in infancy and extensor in childhood
Scarlet fever	Throat culture, ASO titer	Malar flush, circumoral pallor, Pastia lines, desquamation
Insect bites		Check for central punctae
Tinea corporis	KOH smear—long, thin-branched hyphae	
Granuloma annulare		Lack of scale distinguishes from tinea corporis; no epidermal component
Hypopigmented		
Molluscum contagiosum		Pearly papule with central umbilication containing easily expressed white cheesy core
Lichen nitidus		Check penis for grouped lichenoid papules
Lichen striatus, linear lichen planus, epidermal nevus	Skin biopsy	Linear
Violaceous		
Lichen planus		Purple pruritic polygonal papules

Nonblanching

Meningococcemia, sepsis	Blood, cerebrospinal fluid (CSF) culture; gram-stain lesion	Check conjunctivae for hemorrhage
Gonococcemia, SBE	Blood, throat, cervical, rectal cultures	Check for heart murmur, arthritis, tenosynovitis
Henoch-Schönlein purpura†	Stool guaiac, urinalysis, skin biopsy	Abdominal pain, arthritis; crops of lesions
Mastocytosis (urticaria pigmentosa)†	Skin biopsy—mast cells	Wheal and flare on stroking
Letterer-Siwe disease	Skin biopsy—histiocytes	Distinguish from seborrheic dermatitis
Leukemia cutis/lymphoma	Skin biopsy—atypical leukemic infiltrate	Lymphoma, especially Hodgkin disease, may be pruritic
Neuroblastoma, TORCH infection, leukemia	Skin biopsy	"Blueberry muffin" baby

Vesicles

Miliaria crystallina		Superficial
Tinea pedis	KOH scraping of vesicle roof—hyphae	
Herpes simplex; herpes zoster	Tzanck preparation—multinucleated giant cells; viral culture to distinguish simplex from zoster	Grouped vesicles on an erythematous base; simplex labialis, progenitalis, whitlow—zoster usually linear and dermatomal
Contact dermatitis	Patch testing	Sharp borders, linear arrays, bizarre patterns, asymmetrical
Varicella		Crops in various stages—macule, papule, vesicle, pustule, and cyst
Coxsackievirus hand, foot, and mouth disease	Throat culture—coxsackievirus A16, 5, and 10	May be recurrent
Flea bites		Treat pet

Continued.

Laboratory studies and characteristics of skin lesions in children with a rash—cont'd

Diagnosis or differential diagnosis	Laboratory studies	Comments
Bullae		
Bullous disease of childhood	Skin biopsy for hematoxylin and eosin (H&E) stain and immunofluorescence	Refer to dermatologist to rule out bullous pemphigoid and dermatitis herpetiformis
Bullous impetigo	Culture blister fluid for phage group II *S. aureus*	
Pustules		
Erythema toxicum neonatorum	Wright stain of pustule—eosinophils	Pustule in center on erythematous macule
Transient neonatal pustular melanosis	Gram stain of pustule—sterile with PMNs	Hyperpigmented macules; superficial desquamation
Candidiasis	KOH smear of scale or pustule—budding yeast and pseudohyphae	
Folliculitis	Gram stain—staphylococcal or sterile	Follicular, i.e., hair shaft central in pustule; pseudomonas causes hot tub folliculitis
Plaques		
Psoriasis		Well-demarcated erythematous plaque with adherent scale; check family history, arthritis
Acute urticaria	Eosinophil count, throat culture for streptococci, HB$_5$AG	Erythematous, edematous plaque, drug history, food history (shellfish)
Nummular eczema		Papules and vesicles grouped into plaques

*May be popular in parts.
†May be edematous.

Causes of shock in the young infant

Cardiac

Hypoplastic left heart syndrome
Coarctation of the aorta
Myocarditis
Arrhythmia

Infectious

Bacterial meningitis
Urinary tract sepsis
Herpes (meningitis and sepsis)
Streptococcal sepsis

Metabolic

Hypoglycemia
Inborn errors of metabolism

Traumatic

Child abuse
Occult CNS hemorrhage

Surgical

Bowel obstruction
Occult blood loss

See *Primary Pediatric Care,* ed 3, p. 1765.

Features of staphylococcal impetigo versus
streptococcal pyoderma

	Staphylococcal impetigo		Streptococcal pyoderma
Feature	Honey crusted	Bullous	
Most common location	Face	Trunk	Extremities (usually lower)
Nature of early lesion	Vesicle	Bulla	Pustule
Appearance of crust	Honey colored	Thin, brown, varnishlike	Thick, usually brown
Depth of lesion	Superficial	Superficial	Deep
Appearance when crust is removed	Shallow, glistening erosion	Shallow, glistening erosion	Ulcer
Surrounding erythema	None to minimal	None to minimal	Moderate to marked
History of preceding trauma	No	No	Yes
Other nomenclature	Impetigo	Bullous impetigo	Impetigo, nonbullous impetigo, ecthyma

See *Primary Pediatric Care,* ed 3, p. 1203.

Soiling, retentive and nonretentive

Differentiation of retentive soiling from nonretentive soiling

	Retentive soiling	Nonretentive soiling
History		
Symptoms of constipation	Yes	No
Interval	Many times per day	Once per day
Size	Small	Normal
Consistency	Loose	Normal
Previous need for laxatives, suppositories, or enemas	Yes	No
Examination		
Abdominal mass	Yes	No
Abdominal distention	Often	No
Anal canal	Sometimes full	Empty
Rectum	Packed	Normal

See *Primary Pediatric Care*, ed 3, p. 722.

Classification of sprains and strains

	Sprains	Strains
Grade 1	Minimal tearing of ligament No instability of joint End point present on testing of ligament integrity	Microscopic disruptions of musculotendinous unit No defect on physical examination
Grade 2	Appreciable tearing of ligament (5%-99% of fibers disrupted) with moderate joint instability Testing of instability causes pain End point present on testing of ligament integrity	Some tearing of musculotendinous unit Partial loss of function on examination
Grade 3	Complete tear of ligament with absolute joint instability Testing stability of joint causes little pain No clear end point on testing of ligament integrity	Complete rupture of musculotendinous unit May have little pain after a few minutes but dramatic initial sensation of injury

See *Primary Pediatric Care,* ed 3, p. 1606.

Features of stomatitis by category

Type	Organism	Location in mouth	Appearance of lesion	Time to healing	Associated features	Recurrence
Acute primary herpetic gingivostomatitis	HSV1	Anywhere, especially anterior mucosa	Vesicles on red base	7-10 days	Fever, pain, cervical adenopathy, anorexia, dehydration	As cold sores
Herpangina	Enteroviruses, especially coxsackie A4	Posterior, especially soft palate	Small, gray-white vesicles	3-5 days	Mild pain, fever	None
Hand, foot, and mouth disease	Enteroviruses, especially coxsackie A16	Posterior	Small vesicles erode to small ulcers	7 days	Ulcers painful, papular or vesicular rash on palms and soles, fever common	None
Acute necrotizing ulcerative gingivitis (trench mouth)	Oral spirochetes and fusiform bacilli	Gingiva	Red swelling of gums progressing to ulcers with necrotic, gray pseudomembrane	Variable, depends on treatment	Fever, malaise, foul breath	Possible
Aphthous stomatitis						
Minor	Unknown or none	Tongue, labial, and buccal mucosa	Ulcers <1 cm diameter, round or oral, yellow-gray with red halo	7-14 days	Groups of one to five lesions	Common
Major	Unknown or none	Any part of mucosa, especially lips, soft palate, tonsillar pillars	Ulcers >1 cm diameter, deeper than minor	Up to 6 weeks	Submucosal scarring	Common
Herpetiform	Unknown or none	Any part, especially anterior mouth and tongue	Multiple (up to 100) vesicles 1-2 mm diameter	7-10 days	Vesicles may coalesce to small ulcers	Common

See *Primary Pediatric Care*, ed 3, p. 1619.

Differential diagnosis of syncope

Neurocardiogenic

Vasovagal/vasodepressor
episodes
Breath-holding spells
Cyanotic
Pallid infantile syncope

Psychophysiological

Hyperventilation
Hysteria/conversion reaction

Neurological factors

Generalized tonic-clonic
seizure
Atonic seizures
Complex partial seizures
Migraine
Trauma/concussion
Narcolepsy

Cardiac

Structural abnormalities
Aortic stenosis
Idiopathic hypertrophic
subaortic stenosis
Left atrial myxoma
Tetralogy of Fallot
Pulmonic stenosis
Primary pulmonary
hypertension

Arrhythmia
Bradycardia
Sick sinus syndrome
Atrioventricular block
Ventricular tachycardia/
fibrillation
Myocarditis/pericarditis
Intoxication/medication
Congenital heart disease
Postoperative cardiac surgery
Prolonged QT syndrome
Ischemic heart disease
Supraventricular tachycardia
Wolff-Parkinson-White syn-
drome
Caffeine/stress

Orthostatic

Hypovolemia
Postural hypotension
Medications

Metabolic

Hypoglycemia
Anemia

Miscellaneous

Cough
Swallowing
Micturition
Pregnancy

See *Primary Pediatric Care,* ed 3, p. 1129.

Differential diagnosis of abdominal and pelvic tumors in infants and children

Tumor*	Age	Clinical signs	Laboratory findings
Wilms	Preschool	Unilateral flank mass, aniridia, hemihypertrophy	Hematuria
Neuroblastoma	Preschool	GI/GU obstruction, raccoon eyes, myoclonus-opsoclonus, diarrhea, skin nodules (infants)	Increased VMA; increased HVA; increased ferritin; stippled calcification in mass
Non-Hodgkin lymphoma	>1 yr	Intussusception in >2-year-old	Increased urate
Rhabdomyosarcoma	All	GI/GU obstruction, sarcoma botryoides, vaginal bleeding, paratesticular mass	
Germ cell/teratoma	Preschool, teens	Girls: abdominal pain, vaginal bleeding	Increased HCG; increased AFP
		Boys: testicular mass, new-onset "hydrocele"	
		Sacrococcygeal mass/dimple	
Hepatoblastoma	Birth-3 yr	Large, firm liver	Increased AFP
Hepatoma	School age, teens	Large, firm liver; hepatitis B, cirrhosis	Increased AFP

AFP, Alpha-fetoprotein; *GI*, gastrointestinal; *GU*, genitourinary; *HCG*, human chorionic gonadotropin; *HVA*, homovanilic acid; *VMA*, vanillylmandelic acid.
*Other causes: constipation, splenomegaly, hydronephrosis, kidney cyst, and full bladder.

See *Primary Pediatric Care*, ed 3, p. 1217.

Differential diagnosis of head and neck tumors in infants and children

Tumor*	Age	Clinical signs	Laboratory findings
Non-Hodgkin lymphoma	>1 yr	Lymphadenopathy—NR to antibiotics; immunodeficiency; EBV (in Africa)	Increased urate
Hodgkin disease	>10 yr	Lymphadenopathy—NR to antibiotics; weight loss, night sweats, fever, pruritus	Increased ESR
Rhabdomyosarcoma	All	Orbital mass; hoarseness; persistent otitis, sinusitis	
Neuroblastoma	Preschool	Heterochromia iridis, Horner syndrome, myoclonus-opsoclonus, raccoon eyes, skin nodules (infants)	Increased HVA in urine; increased VMA in urine; calcification
Retinoblastoma	Preschool	Cat's eye reflex, strabismus, family history	Calcification

EBV, Epstein-Barr virus; *ESR*, sedimentation rate; *HVA*, homovanillic acid; *NR*, no response; *VMA*, vanillylmandelic acid.
*Other causes: infectious lymphadenopathy, histiocytosis, Caffey disease, acquired immunodeficiency syndrome.

See *Primary Pediatric Care*, ed 3, p. 1219.

Differential diagnosis of malignant tumors involving the extremities

Tumor*	Age	Clinical signs	Laboratory findings
Ewing sarcoma	≥5 yr	Pain, swelling; GU/skeletal anomaly; weight loss, fever; malaise (metabolic)	"Onion skin" on roentgenogram
Osteogenic sarcoma	Teens	Pain, swelling; familial retinoblastoma; prior radiation to bone; Paget disease	Codman triangle (cortical elevation, new bone formation); "sunburst" ossification of soft tissue; soft tissue mass; elevated alkaline phosphatase level
Lymphoma	All	Pain	
Fibrosarcoma	Infants, teens	Painless mass; prior radiation; plastic implant	
Rhabdomyosarcoma	All	Mass	
Synovial sarcoma	Teens	Mass	Calcification (40%)

*Other causes: trauma, bone cysts, osteomyelitis.

See *Primary Pediatric Care*, ed 3, p. 1226.

Differential diagnosis of mediastinal tumors in infants and children

Tumor*	Age	Clinical signs	Laboratory findings
Non-Hodgkin lymphoma	All	Cough, respiratory distress, anterior mediastinal mass, immunodeficiency syndrome	Increased urate; malignant effusion
Hodgkin disease	>10 yr	Middle mediastinum lymphadenopathy—NR to antibiotics; weight loss, night sweats, fever, pruritus	Increased ESR; increased copper
Neuroblastoma	Preschool	Posterior mediastinum; heterochromia iridis, myoclonus-opsoclonus, raccoon eyes, skin nodules (infants)	Increased HVA; increased VMA; calcification
Thymoma	>10 yr	Anterior mediastinum, myasthenia gravis, red cell aplasia, hypogammaglobulinemia	
Germ cell/teratoma	All	Anterior mediastinum (rarely, posterior mediastinum), cough, wheeze, dyspnea	Increased AFP; increased HCG

AFP, Alpha-fetoprotein; *ESR*, sedimentation rate; *HCG*, human chorionic gonadotropin; *HVA*, homovanillic acid; *VMA*, vanillylmandelic acid.
*Other causes: infection, bronchogenic cysts, aneurysms, lipoid tumors, thoracic meningocele.

See *Primary Pediatric Care*, ed 3, p. 1219.

Conditions associated with umbilical hernias

Chromosomal anomalies

Trisomy 13/15
Trisomy 18
Trisomy 21

Metabolic disorders

Hypothyroidism
Mucolipidosis III (pseudo-Hurler syndrome)
Mucopolysaccharidoses
    Type 1 (Hurler syndrome)
    Type 2 (Hunter syndrome)
    Type 4 (Morquio syndrome)

Dysmorphic syndromes

Aarskog syndrome
Beckwith-Wiedemann syndrome
Fetal hydantoin syndrome
Marfan syndrome
Opitz syndrome
Weaver syndrome

From Curry CJR, Honore L, Boyd E: The ventral wall of the trunk. In Stevenson RE, Hall JG, Goodman RM, editors: *Human malformations and related anomalies*, vol 2, New York, 1993, Oxford University Press.

See *Primary Pediatric Care,* ed 3, p. 1639.

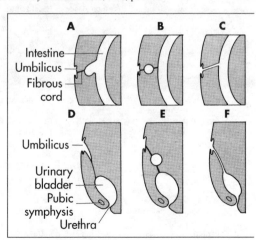

Embryonic umbilical remnants. **A,** Meckel diverticulum. **B,** Enterocystoma. **C,** Enteric (viteline) fistula. **D,** Urachal sinus. **E,** Urachal cyst. **F** Urachal fistula.

See *Primary Pediatric Care,* ed 3, p. 1637.

Causes of vaginal discharge in prepubertal girls

Irritative (bubble baths, sand)
Poor perineal hygiene
Foreign body
Associated systemic illness (group A streptococci, chickenpox)
Infections
    Escherichia coli with foreign body
    Shigella organisms
    Yersinia organisms
Infections (consider sexual abuse)
    Chlamydia trachomatis
    Neisseria gonorrhoeae
    Trichomonas vaginalis
Tumor (rare)

See *Primary Pediatric Care*, ed 3, p. 1144.

Causes of diffuse wheezing

Location	Pathological or anatomical cause	Clinical diagnosis	Type of wheeze generated
Trachea	Loss of airway wall rigidity	Laryngotracheomalacia	Generalized, coarse
	Airway inflammation	Tracheobronchitis, bacterial tracheitis	Generalized, coarse to fine
Bronchi	Less airway wall rigidity	Bronchomalacia	Localized, fine
	Foreign body	Aspirated foreign body	Localized, fine
	Inflammation and mucous obstruction	Bronchiectasis	Localized, fine, bubbly
	Extrinsic compression	Mediastinal tumor or nodes	Localized, coarse
	Airway and elastic tissue destruction	Emphysema	Generalized, fine
	Inflammation	Bronchitis	Generalized, fine
Bronchioles	Inflammation and mucous obstruction	Bronchiolitis	Unusual—generalized, fine, but occasionally localized with mucous obstruction
	Airway wall edema, smooth muscle hypertrophy	Asthma	Same as for bronchiolitis
	Peribronchial edema	Congestive heart failure	Diffuse, fine
	Peribronchial hemorrhage	Hemosiderosis	Focal or diffuse, fine

See *Primary Pediatric Care*, ed 3, p. 1159.

Differential diagnosis of diffuse wheezing by age group

Age group	Acute	Chronic or recurrent
Infants	Infection (bronchiolitis), including tuberculosis and opportunistic infection in immuno-suppressed patients Congestive heart failure Asthma	Tracheomalacia Cystic fibrosis Tracheoesophageal malformations Vascular ring Tracheal stenosis Congenital lobar emphysema Diaphragmatic hernia Bronchopulmonary dysplasia Gastroesophageal reflux Aspiration pneumonitis Extrinsic compression of airway by tumors (e.g., neuroblastoma) Visceral larva migrans Histiocytosis Hemosiderosis Asthma
Children and adolescents	Infection Foreign body Asthma	Foreign body Asthma Allergic bronchopulmonary aspergillosis Cystic fibrosis Ciliary dysmotility syndromes Tumors, lymph nodes Alpha-1-antitrypsin deficiency Sarcoidosis Vocal cord dysfunction Psychogenic causes

See *Primary Pediatric Care,* ed 3, p. 1159.

Diagnostic Approach

Relationship of chronological age (CA), height age (HA), and bone age (BA) with suggested diagnoses

Relationship of CA, HA, and BA	Suggested diagnoses
HA < BA; BA = CA	Genetic short stature, chondrodystrophies, trisomy 21, gonadal dysgenesis (XO), trisomy 13, Cockayne syndrome, leprechaunism, Seckel syndrome, intra-uterine infection, maternal drugs, storage diseases
HA = BA; BA < CA	Normal variant, constitutional delay, familial trait, mild malnutrition, metabolic or other chronic illness
BA < HA; BA < CA	If marked, hypothyroidism; if moderate, hypopituitarism or malnutrition

See *Primary Pediatric Care,* ed 3, p. 951.

Age: chronological, height, and bone

Laboratory evaluation of macrocytic anemias

Diagnosis	Laboratory test	Expected result
Vitamin B_{12} deficiency	Blood film	Macroovalocytes, Howell-Jolly bodies; nucleated RBC and hypersegmented granulocytes
	Serum vitamin B_{12}	Low <100 pg/mL
	Bone marrow examination	Megaloblastic erythroid and granulocyte precursors
Folic acid deficiency	Blood film	Same as above
	Serum folate	Low <3 ng/mL
	RBC folate	Low <160 ng/mL
	Bone marrow examination	Same as above

From Segel GB: *Pediatr Rev* 10:77, 1988.

Anemia, macrocytic

See *Primary Pediatric Care,* ed 3, p. 866.

Laboratory evaluation of hypochromic and microcytic anemias

Diagnosis	Laboratory test	Expected result
Iron deficiency	Serum ferritin	Low <25 μg/L
	Serum iron and total iron-binding capacity	Low/high
	% iron saturation	Low <15%
	Bone marrow iron stores	Absent
	Stool for occult blood	Positive (if gastrointestinal bleeding)
	Urine for blood, hemoglobin, or hemosiderin	Present (if renal loss)
	MCV/RBC ratio	>13
	Blood film	Basophilic stippling
Beta-thalassemia trait	Hemoglobin electrophoresis	Increased A₂ or F hemoglobin
	Biosynthetic beta/alpha-globin chain ratio	<1
	MCV/RBC ratio	<13
	Family studies	Hgb/Hct decreased
		Blood film
		Anisocytosis
		Poikilocytosis
		Basophilic stippling
		MCV <70 fL/cell
Alpha-thalassemia trait	No routine specific test	Normal A₂ hemoglobin
	Family studies	Hgb/Hct normal or slightly decreased
		Blood film
		Anisocytosis
		Poikilocytosis
		MCV <70 fL/cell
	Biosynthetic beta/alpha-globin chain ratio	>1
	Specific genetic probe analysis	Absent genes

See *Primary Pediatric Care,* ed 3, p. 866.

Chronic inflammation		
Nonspecific tests		
Erythrocyte sedimentation rate	Increased
Acute phase reactants	Increased
C-reactive protein	
Fibrinogen	
Haptoglobin	
Serum ferritin	Increased
Serum iron + total iron-binding capacity	Low/low
% iron saturation	Low
Bone marrow iron stores	Increased
Bone marrow sideroblasts	Decreased
Sideroblastic anemia	
Serum ferritin	Increased
Serum iron + total iron-binding capacity	Normal to increased/normal
% iron saturation	High
Bone marrow iron stores	Increased
Bone marrow sideroblasts	Increased sideroblasts plus "ringed" sideroblasts
Lead poisoning	
Blood film	Basophilic stippling
Erythrocyte protoporphyrin	Increased
Blood lead	Increased

From Segel GB: *Pediatr Rev* 10:77, 1988.

MCV, Mean corpuscular volume; *RBC*, red blood cell; *Hgb*, hemoglobin; *Hct*, hematocrit.

Laboratory evaluation of normocytic anemias

Diagnosis	Laboratory test	Expected result
Anemias with low reticulocyte percentage		
Diamond-Blackfan anemia	Bone marrow examination	Decreased erythroid precursors
	Fetal hemoglobin and i antigen	±Increased
	Mean corpuscular volume	±Macrocytosis
Transient erythroblastopenia of childhood	Bone marrow examination	Decreased erythroid precursors
	History	Underlying hemolytic disease
Aplastic crises	Bone marrow examination	Decreased erythroid precursors
	Serology and/or viral culture	Parvovirus
Anemias with high reticulocyte percentage		
Extrinsic		
Autoimmune hemolysis	Blood film	Spherocytes
	Antiglobulin (Coombs) test	Positive
	Complement consumption assay	Positive (used if Coombs test is negative)
	Tests for underlying disease	

See *Primary Pediatric Care*, ed 3, p. 866.

Fragmentation hemolytic anemia	Blood film	Fragmented RBC
	Tests for underlying disease	
Intrinsic		
Membrane disorders	Blood film	Characteristic RBC: spherocytes, stomatocytes, elliptocytes
	Incubated osmotic fragility	Increased fragility if spherocytes present
	Autohemolysis	Increased and corrected by glucose
	Membrane protein-structural analysis (investigational)	Abnormal (e.g., decreased spectrin in spherocytosis)
Hemoglobin disorders	Blood film	Irreversibly sickled cells in severe sickle syndromes: SS-, SC-, or S-thalassemia
		Targeting in CC, also in SS-, SC-, and S-thalassemia
	Hemoglobin electrophoresis	Abnormal hemoglobins
Enzyme disorders G6PD	Screening tests	Positive
	Enzyme assay	Low activity
Pyruvate kinase and other glycolytic defects	Enzyme assay	Low activity

From Segel GB: *Pediatr Rev* 10:77, 1988.

Attention deficit/hyperactivity disorder: diagnostic criteria*

I. Either (A) or (B)

—Lasting 6 months or longer

—Severe enough to be maladaptive and inconsistent with normal development

   (A) Inattention (at least six of the following nine symptoms):

      1. Often fails to give close attention to details or makes careless mistakes in schoolwork, work, or other activities

      2. Often has difficulty sustaining attention in tasks or play activities

      3. Often does not seem to listen when spoken to directly

      4. Often does not follow through on instructions and fails to finish schoolwork, chores, or duties in the work place (not due to oppositional behavior or failure to understand instructions)

      5. Often has difficulty organizing tasks and activities

      6. Often avoids, dislikes, or is reluctant to engage in tasks that require sustained mental effort such as schoolwork or homework

      7. Often loses things necessary for tasks or activities (e.g., toys, school assignments, pencils, books, or tools).

      8. Often is easily distracted by extraneous stimuli

      9. Often is forgetful in daily activities

   (B) Hyperactivity/Impulsivity (at least six of the following nine symptoms):

   Hyperactivity

      1. Often fidgets with hands or feet or squirms in seat

      2. Often leaves seat in classroom or in other situations in which remaining seated is expected

      3. Often runs about or climbs excessively when it is inappropriate (may be limited to subjective feelings of restlessness in older individuals)

      4. Often has difficulty playing or engaging in leisure activities quietly

      5. Often is "on the go" or acts as if "driven by a motor"

      6. Often talks excessively

   Impulsivity

      7. Often blurts out answers before questions have been completed

      8. Often has difficulty waiting for his or her turn

      9. Often interrupts or intrudes on others (e.g., butts into conversations or games)

II. Symptoms (at least some of those noted above) present before 7 years of age

III. Some impaired function in two or more settings (e.g., school, work, and home)

IV. Clear evidence of impairment in social, academic, or occupational functioning

Attention deficit/hyperactivity disorder: diagnostic criteria*—cont'd

V. Symptoms are not exclusively associated with
    Pervasive developmental disorder
    Schizophrenia or other psychoses and are not better
      accounted for by
    Mood disorder
    Anxiety disorder
    Dissociative disorder
    Personality disorder

*From The American Psychiatric Association: *Diagnostic and statistical manual of mental disorders*, ed 4, Washington, DC, 1994, The Association.

See *Primary Pediatric Care*, ed 3, p. 671.

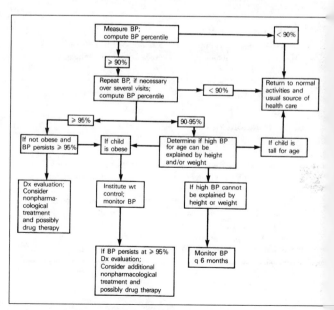

Algorithm for identifying children with high blood pressure. (From Task Force on Blood Pressure Control in Children: *Pediatrics* 79:1, 1987; courtesy Dr. Michael J. Horan.)
See *Primary Pediatric Care*, ed 3, p. 1008.

DSM-IV diagnostic criteria for conduct disorder

A. A repetitive and persistent pattern of behavior in which the basic rights of others or major age-appropriate societal norms or rules are violated, as manifested by the presence of three (or more) of the following criteria in the past 12 months, with at least one criterion present in the past 6 months:

Aggression to people and animals

1. Often bullies, threatens, or intimidates others
2. Often initiates physical fights with others
3. Has used a weapon that can cause serious physical harm to others (e.g., bat, brick, broken bottle, knife, gun)
4. Has been physically cruel to people
5. Has been physically cruel to animals
6. Has stolen while confronting a victim (e.g., mugging, purse snatching, extorting, armed robbery)
7. Has forced someone into sexual activity

Destruction of property

8. Has deliberately engaged in fire-setting with the intention of causing serious damage
9. Has deliberately destroyed others' property (other than by fire-setting)

Deceitfulness or theft

10. Has broken into someone else's house, building, or car
11. Often lies to obtain goods or favors or to avoid obligations (i.e., "cons" others)
12. Has stolen items of nontrivial value without confronting a victim (i.e., shoplifting, but without breaking and entering, or forgery)

Serious violations of rules

13. Often stays out at night despite parental prohibitions, beginning before age 13 years
14. Has run away from home overnight at least twice while living in parental or parental-surrogate home (or once without returning for a lengthy period)
15. Often is truant from school, beginning before age 13 years

B. The disturbance in behavior causes clinically significant impairment in social, academic, or occupational functioning.
C. If the individual is age 18 years or older, criteria are not met for antisocial personality disorder.

See *Primary Pediatric Care,* ed 3, p. 716.

Criteria for diagnosis of conversion symptoms

The symptom has symbolic meaning to the patient.
The patient frequently exhibits characteristic interpersonal behaviors.
Conversion symptoms are more common in girls than boys.
There is a characteristic style of reporting symptoms.
The symptom helps the patient cope with his or her environment
    ("secondary gain").
There often is frequent use of health issues and symptoms in family
    communication.
Symptoms occur at times of stress.
The symptom has a model.
History and physical findings often are inconsistent with anatomical
    and physiological concepts.

From Prazar G: *Pediatr Rev* 8:279, 1987.

See *Primary Pediatric Care,* ed 3, p. 785.

Signs and symptoms of pulmonary exacerbation in cystic fibrosis*

Change in sputum volume, color, and appearance
Deterioration in pulmonary function test results
Increased cough, dyspnea, and tachypnea
New chest examination findings
New chest radiographic findings
Fever
Fatigue
Decreased exercise tolerance
Decreased appetite
Weight loss

*Often insidious onset.

See *Primary Pediatric Care,* ed 3, p. 419.

Signs and symptoms related to degree of dehydration*

	Degree of dehydration		
Parameter	**Mild**	**Moderate**	**Severe**
Weight loss (%)†	3-5 (2-3)	10 (7)	15 (9-12)
Skin color	Pale	Gray	Mottled
Skin turgor	May be normal	Decreased	Tenting
Mucous membranes	Slightly dry	Dry	Dry, parched, collapse of sublingual veins
Eyes	Probably normal	Decreased tears	Sunken, absence of tears, soft globes
CNS	Normal	Irritable	Lethargic
Pulse			
Quality	Strong	Somewhat decreased	Distal pulse not palpable
Rate	Probably normal	Somewhat increased (orthostatic changes)	Markedly tachycardic
Capillary refill	Normal (<2 seconds)	2-4 seconds	>4 seconds
Blood pressure	No change	Orthostatic decrease	Decreased while supine
Urine	Probably normal or slightly decreased volume	Elevated specific gravity, decreased volume	Less than 0.5 ml/kg/hr over past 12-24 hr; may be anuric

*Table is most useful for situations involving isotonic dehydration.
†Percentage of weight loss listed applies to infants younger than 1 year of age. In older children and adults, dehydration becomes more notable with smaller losses of water (these values are listed in parentheses).

See *Primary Pediatric Care,* ed 3, p. 341.

Criteria for the diagnosis of atopic dermatitis

Major criteria (all three must be present)

1. Pruritus
2. Typical morphology and distribution
   a. Facial and extensor involvement during infancy and early childhood
   b. Flexural lichenification and linearity by adolescence
3. Chronic or recurring dermatitis

Minor criteria (two or more must be present)

1. Personal or family history of atopy (e.g., asthma, allergic rhinoconjunctivitis, atopic dermatitis)
2. Immediate skin test reactivity
3. White dermatographism and/or delayed blanch to cholinergic agents
4. Anterior subcapsular cataracts

Associated conditions (four or more must be present)

1. Xerosis/ichthyosis/hyperlinear palms
2. Pityriasis alba
3. Keratosis pilaris
4. Facial pallor/infraorbital darkening
5. Dennie-Morgan fold
6. Elevated serum IgE
7. Keratoconus
8. Nonspecific hand dermatitis
9. Recurring cutaneous infections

See *Primary Pediatric Care,* ed 3, p. 1196.

Evaluation of acute diarrhea

History

1. Length of illness
2. Stools—frequency, looseness (watery versus mushy), and presence of gross blood
3. Oral intake—diet, quantity of fluids and solids taken, and presence of vomiting
4. Associated symptoms—fever, rash, and arthralgia
5. Urine output
6. Contacts with diarrhea or other infectious illness (including day care exposure)

Physical examination

1. Hydration status—moist mucosa, presence of saliva and tears, skin turgor, weight, and vital signs
2. Alertness
3. Infant—vigor of suck

Laboratory

1. Stool culture (as indicated), smear for white blood cells, and evaluation for occult blood
2. Stool ova and parasites and reducing substances (as indicated)
3. Complete blood count (as indicated)
4. If hydration status is in question—blood urea nitrogen (BUN) and serum electrolyte levels
5. Urinalysis
6. If child is lethargic or has had a seizure, culture for sepsis: measure the BUN and serum electrolyte levels and examine and culture the cerebrospinal fluid (as indicated)

See *Primary Pediatric Care,* ed 3, p. 904.

Common features of Down syndrome

May or may not be present:

Head
  Brachycephaly (flat occiput)

Dermatoglyphics
  Increased ulnar loops
  Single flexion crease on fifth finger
  Four-finger sign (simian crease): transverse palmar lines

Eyes
  Brushfield spots (speckling of the iris)
  Inner epicanthal folds
  Upward slanting palpebral fissures (mongolian characteristic)

Face
  Flat appearing
  Low nasal bridge
  Small ears with small or no earlobes

Fingers and toes
  Brachydactyly (short hands and fingers)
  Wide-spaced first and second toes

Heart (commonly congenital defects)
  Endocardial cushion defects
  Ventricular septal defects

Hips and pelvis
  Dysplasia

Neck
  Short
  Superabundant skin at nape

Neuromuscular system
  Absent or diminished Moro reflex
  Muscular hypotonia
  Joint hyperflexibility

Tongue
  Macroglossia
  Excessive protrusion

Potential for:

Increased incidence of leukemia
Increased susceptibility to infection
Increased incidence of duodenal atresia

See *Primary Pediatric Care*, ed 3, p. 1282.

Manifestations of neonatal drug withdrawal

Central nervous system signs

Exaggerated reflexes
Hyperactivity
Hyperirritability (excess crying, high-pitched cry)
Increased muscle tone
Short, nonquiet sleep
Sneezing, hiccups, yawning
Tremors

Respiratory signs

Excess secretions
Tachypnea

Gastrointestinal signs

Abdominal cramps (?)
Diarrhea
Disorganized, poor sucking
Drooling
Hyperphagia
Sensitive gag reflex
Vomiting

Vasomotor signs

Flushing
Stuffy nose
Sudden, circumoral pallor
Sweating

Cutaneous signs

Excoriated buttocks
Facial scratches
Pressure point abrasions

Fever

See *Primary Pediatric Care,* ed 3, p. 563.

Criteria for the diagnosis of eating disorders

Anorexia nervosa

Refusal to maintain body weight at or above a minimally normal weight for age and height (e.g., weight loss leading to maintenance of body weight less than 85% of that expected; or failure to make expected weight gain during period of growth, leading to body weight less than 85% of that expected).

Intense fear of gaining weight or becoming fat, even though underweight.

Disturbance in the way in which one's body weight or shape is experienced, undue influence of body weight or shape on self-evaluation, or denial of seriousness of the current low body weight.

In postmenarcheal females, amenorrhea, i.e., the absence of at least three consecutive menstrual cycles. (A woman is considered to have amenorrhea if her periods occur only following hormone, e.g., estrogen, administration.)

Restricting type: during the current episode of anorexia nervosa, the person has not regularly engaged in binge-eating or purging behavior (i.e., self-induced vomiting or the misuse of laxatives, diuretics, or enemas).

Binge-eating/purging type: during the current episode of anorexia nervosa, the person has regularly engaged in binge-eating or purging behavior (i.e., self-induced vomiting or the misuse of laxatives, diuretics, or enemas).

Bulimia nervosa

Recurrent episodes of binge eating. An episode of binge eating is characterized by both of the following:

> Eating, in a discrete period of time (e.g., within any 2-hour period), an amount of food that is definitely larger than most people would eat during a similar period of time and under similar circumstances

> A sense of lack of control over eating during the episode (e.g., a feeling that one cannot stop eating or control what or how much one is eating)

Recurrent inappropriate compensatory behavior in order to prevent weight gain, such as self-induced vomiting; misuse of laxatives, diuretics, enemas, or other medications; fasting; or excessive exercise.

The binge eating and inappropriate compensatory behaviors both occur, on average, at least twice a week for 3 months.

Self-evaluation is unduly influenced by body shape and weight.

The disturbance does not occur exclusively during episodes of anorexia nervosa.

See *Primary Pediatric Care,* ed 3, p. 792.

Criteria for the diagnosis of eating disorders—cont'd

Bulimia nervosa—cont'd

Purging type: during the current episode of bulimia nervosa, the person has regularly engaged in self-induced vomiting or the misuse of laxatives, diuretics, or enemas.

Nonpurging type: during the current episode of bulimia nervosa, the person has used other inappropriate compensatory behaviors, such as fasting or excessive exercise, but has not regularly engaged in self-induced vomiting or the misuse of laxatives, diuretics, or enemas.

From The American Psychiatric Association: *Diagnostic and statistical manual of mental disorders,* ed 4, Washington, DC, 1994, The Association.

Eating disorders—cont'd

Evaluation of the individual who has facial dysmorphism

1. Describe the dysmorphic facial features
2. Describe any other dysmorphic somatic features
3. Define the growth of the individual in weight, length, and head circumference
4. Define the development of the individual
5. Review the gestational and perinatal history
6. Review the family history
7. Consider laboratory tests
8. Determine if the features fit a recognizable syndrome
9. Discuss the findings with the family

Facial dysmorphism

See *Primary Pediatric Care,* ed 3, p. 947.

Pertinent clinical findings in genetic-metabolic disorders

System	Findings
Neurological	Encephalopathy
	Strokelike episodes
	Macrocephaly
	Developmental delay
	Ataxia
	Choreoathetosis
	Dystonia
	Hypotonia or hypertonia
	Seizures
	Myoclonus
	Deafness
	Brain malformations
Ophthalmological	Cataracts
	Corneal opacities
	Macular cherry red spot
	Lens dislocation
	Retinal pigmentary changes
Respiratory	Tachypnea
	Hyperpnea
Cardiovascular	Cardiomyopathy
	Pericardial effusion
	Rhythm disturbance
	Thrombosis
Abdominal	Hepatomegaly
	Cirrhosis
	Jaundice
	Splenomegaly
	Nephrolithiasis
	Renal Fanconi syndrome
	Renal cysts
	Pancreatitis
Muscular	Hypertrophy
	Myopathy
	Myalgias
	Recurrent myoglobinuria
Skin	Eczematous rash
	Ichthyosis
	Photosensitivity
	Angiokeratomas
Hair	Sparse
	Brittle, dry
Skeletal	Scoliosis
	Kyphosis
	Joint contractures
	Dysostosis multiplex
	Epiphyseal calcifications
Other	Dysmorphic features
	Coarse facial features

See *Primary Pediatric Care,* ed 3, p. 206.

High-risk scenarios for the consideration of metabolic disorders

Clinical picture	Disorders to consider
Acute illness in a previously normal newborn	Aminoacidopathies, organic acidemias, urea cycle defects, galactosemia
Neonatal seizure disorder	Pyridoxine-dependent seizures, nonketotic hyperglycinemia, sulfite oxidase deficiency
Recurrent episodic illness (lethargy, vomiting, ataxia, encephalopathy, strokelike episodes, myopathy, "near miss" SIDS)	Aminoacidopathies, organic acidemias, urea cycle defects, defects in fatty acid metabolism, disorders of carbohydrate metabolism, mitochondrial disorders
Neurological regression	Lysosomal storage disorders, X-linked adrenoleukodystrophy
Chronic, progressive symptomology (poor feeding, poor growth, slow development, neurological and other organ system dysfunction)	Aminoacidopathies, organic acidemias, disorders of carbohydrate metabolism; mitochondrial and peroxisomal diseases

See *Primary Pediatric Care*, ed 3, p. 204.

Initial blood and urine tests for suspected genetic-metabolic disorders

Blood tests	Abnormal finding	Disease
Blood gases, electrolytes	Metabolic acidosis, elevated anion gap	Organic acidemias, maple syrup urine disease, disorders of carbohydrate metabolism, mitochondrial defects
	Respiratory alkalosis	Urea cycle defects
Glucose	Low with ketosis	Disorders of carbohydrate metabolism, organic acidemias
	Low without ketosis	Fatty acid oxidation defects
Ammonia	High	Urea cycle defects, organic acidemias, fatty acid oxidation defects, nongenetic disorders that have significant liver dysfunction
Lactate, pyruvate	High	Disorders of carbohydrate metabolism, respiratory chain defects, severe tissue hypoxia
Uric acid	High	Glycogen storage disorders, fatty acid oxidation defects, organic acidemias
Urea nitrogen	Low	Urea cycle disorders
Liver transaminases	High	Tyrosinemia, galactosemia, hereditary fructose intolerance, fatty acid oxidation defects
Phosphate	Low	Hereditary fructose intolerance, fructose 1,6 diphosphatase deficiency
Creatine kinase	High	Primary carnitine defects, fatty acid oxidation disorders, mitochondrial myopathies, muscular dystrophies
Blood count	Neutropenia, thrombocytopenia	Organic acidemias

Urine tests	Abnormal finding	Disease
Odor (assess by opening a closed container left at room temperature for 3 hours)	Sweaty feet, musty, tomcat urine, maple syrup	Organic acidemias, aminoacidopathies
Ketones—essential test whenever hypoglycemia is documented	Positive	Organic acidemias, maple syrup urine disease, disorders of carbohydrate metabolism
Reducing substances (requires urine glucose determination for interpretation)	Positive with glucose, galactose, fructose	Galactosemia, hereditary fructose intolerance

See *Primary Pediatric Care,* ed 3, p. 207.

Specific laboratory tests for genetic-metabolic disorders

Type	Diseases
Blood	
Quantitative plasma amino acids	Aminoacidopathies, abnormalities also found in organic acidemias and disorders of carbohydrate metabolism
Carnitine levels (total, free, and esterified), acylcarnitine profile	Disorders of fatty acid metabolism
Very long chain fatty acids, plasmalogens, phytanic acid	Peroxisomal disorders
Urine	
Quantitative amino acids	Specific amino acid transport defects, Fanconi syndrome
Organic acids	Organic acidemias
Oligosaccharide thin layer chromatography	Lysosomal disorders of glycoprotein degradation
Screens (ferric chloride, dinitrophenylhydrazine, sulfite oxidase, mucopolysaccharide spot)	Aminoacidopathies, organic acidemias, mucopolysaccharidoses (frequent false positives and negatives)
Spinal fluid	
Amino acids (glycine)	Nonketotic hyperglycinemia (requires simultaneous plasma amino acids)
Enzyme assays	
Blood, skin, or other tissue	Required for diagnosis of all lysosomal storage disorders, definitive diagnosis of most metabolic disorders

Note: In the event the child dies before a definitive diagnosis is made, a small piece of muscle and liver should be quick frozen and held at −70°. A skin biopsy for cultured fibroblasts should be obtained premortem.

See *Primary Pediatric Care,* ed 3, p. 207.

Presenting symptoms and signs of heart failure

Diaphoresis   Tachypnea
Poor feeding   Tachycardia, gallop rhythm
Failure to thrive   Murmur
Apnea   Rales, rhonchi, wheezes
Peripheral edema   Hepatomegaly

See *Primary Pediatric Care,* ed 3, p. 1713.

Pathogens in HIV-infected children

Organism	Syndrome	Method of diagnosis	Treatment	Comments
Pneumocystis carinii	Pneumonia	Pneumocysts seen on special stains of respiratory specimen or tissue	TMP-SMX (20 mg/kg TMP component/day IV or PO) or pentamidine isethionate (4 mg/kg/day IV or IM)	Toxic effects of therapy are common; treat for 21 days, relapses are common, prophylaxis may be beneficial
Toxoplasma gondii	Brain abscess	Brain scans; biopsy	Sulfadiazine and pyrimethamine (PO)	Toxic effects of therapy are common; use folinic acid; lifelong therapy is required to prevent relapse
Cryptosporidium sp.	Gastroenteritis	Stool examination (special procedure); biopsy	Best therapy is not known; supportive	Chronic infection
Candida sp.	Thrush, esophagitis	Wet mount or gram stain of lesions (thrush); esophagoscopy and biopsy (esophagus)	Clotrimazole, ketoconazole, fluconazole, amphotericin B	Relapses are common; consider maintenance
Cryptococcus sp.	Meningitis, fungemia, pneumonia	Cryptococcal antigen tests on blood, CSF; culture of blood, respiratory specimen, CSF; India ink test on CSF	Amphotericin B	Flucytosine can be used if tolerated; chronic suppressive therapy is required to prevent relapse

See *Primary Pediatric Care,* ed 3, p. 1178.

Organism	Manifestations	Diagnosis	Treatment	Comments
Cytomegalovirus	Chorioretinitis, pneumonitis, hepatitis, colitis, esophagitis, encephalitis, disseminated (including adrenals)	Ophthalmological examination (retinitis); tissue biopsy; culture (urine, sputum, buffy coat)	Gancyclovir	Relapses occur after therapy; suppressive regimen is required; isolation of virus does not alone provide diagnosis
Herpes simplex virus	Stomatitis, perianal infection	Tzanck preparation; culture	Acyclovir (750 mg/m^2/day IV, can treat PO)	Recurrences are frequent; chronic suppressive therapy may be needed
Varicella-zoster virus	Primary varicella, local or disseminated zoster	Tzanck preparation; culture	Acyclovir (1500 mg/m^2/day IV)	Chronic or relapsing zoster lesions occur; indications for and effectiveness of oral therapy are not clear
Mycobacterium avium/intracellulare	Disseminated infection (blood, bone marrow, liver, spleen, GI tract, nodes)	Acid-fast blood culture; acid-fast stain or culture of tissue or fluid specimen	Clarithromycin	Drugs used have included ansamycin, clofazimine, ethambutol, amikacin, rifampin, isoniazid, and ethionamide, but their efficacy has not been documented

Modified from Falloon J et al: *J Pediatr* 114:17, 1989.
TMP-SMX, Trimethoprim-sulfamethoxazole.

High-risk historical factors for HIV infection

Women of childbearing age

Intravenous drug use
Multiple sexual partners
Blood transfusions before 1985
A sexual partner with any of the following characteristics:
· Known infection with HIV
· Bisexual practices
· History of IV drug use
· Hemophilia
· Blood transfusions before 1985

Neonatal and early childhood

Prematurity
Low birth weight
Recurrent oral thrush
Failure to thrive
Recurrent fevers
Chronic diarrhea
Recurrent infections
Opportunistic infections
Blood transfusions
Sexual abuse

Adolescents

IV drug abuse
Tattoos
Sexual practices
· Number of partners
· Homosexual preference
· Bisexual preference
· Contraceptive methods

See *Primary Pediatric Care*, ed 3, p. 1172.

Criteria for identifying pathological hyperbilirubinemia in newborns

Clinical jaundice in the first 24 hours of life
Total serum bilirubin concentrations increasing by more than 5 mg/dl (85 μmol/l/day)
Total serum bilirubin concentrations exceeding 12.9 mg/dl (221 μmol/l) in full-term infants or 15 mg/dl (257 μmol/l) in premature infants
Direct (conjugated) serum bilirubin concentration exceeding 1.5 to 2 mg/dl (25 to 34 μmol/l)
Clinical jaundice persisting for more than 1 week in full-term infants or 2 weeks in premature infants

See *Primary Pediatric Care*, ed 3, p. 539.

Assessment of severe hypertension in children

Present or past medical history of | Suggests

Present or past medical history of	Suggests
Headache, visual disturbance, irritability, abdominal pain (in young child)	Malignant or accelerated hypertension
Drug use	Drug-induced hypertension
Umbilical artery catheter	Renovascular hypertension
Sore throat	Glomerulonephritis
Recurrent cough, shortness of breath	Preexisting congestive heart failure, pulmonary edema
Weight loss or gain	Hyperthyroidism, pheochromocytoma, Cushing syndrome, congestive heart failure, renal failure, nephrosis
Palpitations, flushing, diarrhea	Hyperthyroidism, pheochromocytoma
Bloody diarrhea	Hemolytic-uremic syndrome
Purpuric-petechial rash	Vasculitis syndrome

Physical findings of

Physical findings of	
Thin general appearance	Hyperthyroidism, pheochromocytoma
Obese general appearance (truncal)	Cushing syndrome
Blood pressure normal or much lower in lower extremity than upper extremity	Aortic coarctation
Edema	Congestive heart failure, renal failure, nephrosis
Skin	
Ash-leaf spots	Tuberous sclerosis
Café-au-lait spots	Neurofibromatosis
Rash	Vasculitis
Pyoderma	Glomerulonephritis
HEENT	
Rounded (moon) facies	Cushing syndrome
Proptosis, goiter	Hyperthyroidism
Papilledema	Intracranial mass or hemorrhage
Heart	
Cardiomegaly	Congestive heart failure or long-standing hypertension
Murmur	Aortic coarctation
Abdomen	
Mass involving flank(s)	Tumor (Wilms, neuroblastoma) obstructive uropathy, polycystic kidney disease
Bruit	Renal artery stenosis
Ambiguous genitalia	Virilizing adrenal hyperplasia

See *Primary Pediatric Care*, ed 3, p. 1715.

Symptoms and signs of hypothyroidism

Congenital hypothyroidism

Facial edema
Large posterior fontanelle
 (>0.5 cm)
Rectal temperature below 95° F
 (35° C)
Decreased stooling (less than one
 stool per day)
Prolonged hyperbilirubinemia
 (bilirubin above 10 mg/dl after
 3 days of age)
Respiratory distress in a term in-
 fant
Umbilical hernia
Birth weight above 4000 g
Macroglossia
Bradycardia (pulse below 100
 beats/min)
Feeding problems and lethargy
Cutaneous mottling, vasomotor
 instability
Hoarse cry
Hirsute forehead

Juvenile hypothyroidism

Growth retardation (below 4
 cm/yr)
Delayed bone maturation
Delayed dental development and
 tooth eruption
Onset of puberty: usually de-
 layed; rarely precocious
Myopathy and muscular hyper-
 trophy
Menstrual disorders
Galactorrhea
Increased skin pigmentation
Physical and mental turpor
Pale, gray, cool, mottled, thick-
 ened, coarse skin
Constipation
Coarse, dry brittle hair

See *Primary Pediatric Care,* ed 3, p. 1358.

Laboratory screening tests for immunodeficiency syndromes

1. Antibody deficiency syndromes
   a. Immunoglobulin levels (normal level is age related)
   b. Isohemagglutinin titers
   c. Specific antibody titers (i.e., polio and tetanus)
   d. HIV antibody
2. Leukocyte deficiency syndromes
   a. Granulocyte count (should have 1500 or more granulocytes)
   b. Stained peripheral smear (look at granule size)
   c. Nitroblue tetrazolium (NBT) test
3. Complement deficiency syndromes
   a. Total hemolytic complement
   b. C3 level (radial diffusion kits available)
4. T cell deficiency syndromes
   a. Chest roentgenogram for thymus shadow
   b. Skin test using *Candida* organisms, mumps, SK-SO, and teta-
      nus toxoid
   c. Total lymphocyte count (should have 1500 or more)
   d. HIV antibody

See *Primary Pediatric Care,* ed 3, p. 1093.

Evaluation of children who have recurrent infections

Category A: generally well child*

1. Normal growth and development
2. Usual illness with common viruses
3. Infections usually of skin and upper respiratory tract, such as furunculosis, otitis media, and rhinitis
4. Infection usually with common pathogens such as respiratory viruses, *Staphylococcus*, and *Streptococcus*
5. Periods of complete wellness
6. Chest roentgenogram usually normal
7. Palpable lymph nodes and normal-to-enlarged tonsils

Category B: child who has specific signs and symptoms that may indicate immunodeficiency or another chronic illness†

1. Failure to thrive
2. Severe disease with common viruses such as chickenpox and measles
3. More than one *serious infection*, such as meningitis, pneumonia, bone and joint infection, or bacteremia
4. May be infected with organisms that usually are of low virulence in the normal host (e.g., *Serratia, Klebsiella, Pseudomonas, Proteus*)
5. Few periods when child is completely well
6. Chest roentgenogram usually abnormal
7. Physical signs such as the following:
   a. Rales or wheezing
   b. Chronic eczema and alopecia
   c. Small tonsils and nonpalpable lymph nodes
   d. Chronic blepharitis
   e. Opacified sinuses
   f. Clubbing of fingers
   g. Nasal polyps
   h. Chronic mucopurulent nasal or postnasal drainage
8. Chronic diarrhea or stools characteristic of malabsorption
9. Frequent fever

*Children in this category usually need to have their acute infections (e.g., otitis media) treated and their *parents reassured* that generally they are well. Drawing specific attention to each of the items of information that caused them to be put in this category is very comforting to most parents.

†Any one of the items in this category may indicate a need for systematic laboratory evaluation that is specifically designed to *follow the clues*. It is painful, expensive, and reckless to try to rule out every possibility in the differential diagnosis with a "laboratory shotgun" approach.

See *Primary Pediatric Care*, ed 3, p. 1090.

Symptoms and signs of acute and chronic increased intracranial pressure

Infants
Acute

Irritability
Poor feeding/emesis
Split sutures (especially lambdoidal)
Bulging fontanelle
Altered mental status
Seizures
Parinaud sign (upgaze paresis)

Chronic

Irritability
Poor feeding/emesis
Increased head circumference
Bulging fontanelle
Split sutures (especially lambdoidal)
Apparent developmental arrest or regression
Parinaud sign

Children
Acute

Severe, acute headache
Seizures
Emesis
Rapidly deteriorating mental status
Decerebrate/decorticate posture
Focal neurological deficits
+/− Papilledema
Pupillary abnormalities
Autonomic dysfunction (Cushing triad)

Chronic

Chronic, progressive headache
Seizures
Early morning emesis
Change in school performance
Altered mental status
Cranial neuropathy (e.g., sixth cranial nerve palsy)
Focal neurological deficits
Papilledema
Visual changes

See *Primary Pediatric Care,* ed 3, p. 1726.

Diagnostic criteria for Kawasaki disease

A. Principal symptoms (At least five of the following six items should be satisfied for diagnosis.)
   1. Fever of unknown cause lasting 5 days or more
   2. Bilateral congestion of ocular conjunctivae
   3. Changes of lips and oral cavity
      a. Dryness, redness, and fissuring of lips
      b. Protuberance of tongue papillae (strawberry tongue)
      c. Diffuse reddening of oral and pharyngeal mucosa
   4. Changes of peripheral extremities
      a. Reddening of palms and soles (initial stage)
      b. Indurative edema (initial stage)
      c. Membranous desquamation from fingertips (convalescent stage)
   5. Polymorphous exanthema of body trunk without vesicles or crusts
   6. Acute nonpurulent swelling of cervical lymph nodes of 1.5 cm or more in diameter

B. Other significant symptoms or findings
   1. Carditis, especially myocarditis or pericarditis
   2. Diarrhea
   3. Arthralgia or arthritis
   4. Proteinuria and increase of leukocytes in urine sediment
   5. Changes in blood tests
      a. Leukocytosis with shift to the left
      b. Slight decrease in erythrocyte and hemoglobin levels
      c. Increased sedimentation rate
      d. Elevated C-reactive protein (CRP)
      e. Increased beta-2-globulin
      f. Thrombocytosis
      g. Negative antistreptolysin titer (ASO)
   6. Changes occasionally observed
      a. Aseptic meningitis
      b. Mild jaundice or slight increase of serum transaminase
      c. Swelling of gallbladder

See *Primary Pediatric Care*, ed 3, p. 1390.

Risk factors for coronary artery aneurysms in Kawasaki disease

Risk very increased

Fever lasts longer than 14 days
Biphasic fever pattern*†
Biphasic pattern of skin rash
Maximum WBC count ≥30,000
Maximum ESR (mm/hr) ≥101
Time until normalization of ESR or CRP ≥30 days of illness
Biphasic elevation of ESR or CRP†
Increased Q/R ratio in leads II, III, aV_F >0.3
Symptoms of myocardial infarction

Risk increased

Male sex
Age at onset under 1 year
Hemoglobin ≤10 g/dl† and RBC count ≤3.5 million
Maximum WBC count >26,000
Maximum ESR (mm/hr) >50
Cardiomegaly
Arrhythmia
Recurrence of disease

*Separated by afebrile period of 48 hours or longer.
†Causes other than Kawasaki disease must be ruled out.

See *Primary Pediatric Care,* ed 3, p. 1394.

Factors associated with increased risk for childhood leukemia

Familial predisposition

Twin of a patient with leukemia
Sibling of a patient with leukemia

Genetic factors

Down syndrome
Fanconi anemia
Bloom syndrome
Ataxia telangiectasia
Congenital hypogammaglobulinemia
Wiskott-Aldrich syndrome
Neurofibromatosis
Poland syndrome
Klinefelter syndrome
Schwachman syndrome

Environmental exposure

Viral infection
Ionizing radiation (atomic bomb and nuclear accidents)
Therapeutic radiation (ankylosing spondylitis, thymic enlargement)
Prenatal diagnostic radiation exposure
Certain drugs (benzene, alkylating agents)
Modified from Neglia JP, Robinson LL: *Pediatr Clin North Am* 35:675, 1988.

See *Primary Pediatric Care,* ed 3, p. 1399.

Manifestations of Lyme disease by stage*

| System† | Early infection | | Late infection: persistent (stage 3) |
	Localized (stage 1)	Disseminated (stage 2)	
Skin	Erythema chronicum migrans	Secondary annular lesions, malar rash, diffuse erythema or urticaria, evanescent lesions, lymphocytoma	Acrodermatitis chronica atrophicans, localized scleroderma-like lesions
Musculoskeletal system		Migratory pain in joints, tendons, bursae, muscle, bone, brief arthritis attacks, myositis,‡ osteomyelitis,‡ panniculitis‡	Prolonged arthritis attacks, chronic arthritis, peripheral enthesopathy, periostitis or joint subluxations below lesions of acrodermatitis
Neurological system		Meningitis, cranial neuritis, Bell palsy, motor or sensory radiculoneuritis, subtle encephalitis, mononeuritis multiplex, myelitis,‡ chorea,‡ cerebellar ataxia‡	Chronic encephalomyelitis, spastic parapareses, ataxic gait, subtle mental disorders, chronic axonal polyradiculopathy, dementia‡

Continued.

See *Primary Pediatric Care,* ed 3, p. 1415.

Manifestations of Lyme disease by stage*—cont'd

| System† | Early infection | | Late infection: persistent (stage 3) |
	Localized (stage 1)	Disseminated (stage 2)	
Lymphatic system	Regional lymphadenopathy	Regional or generalized lymphadenopathy, splenomegaly	
Heart		Atrioventricular nodal block, myopericarditis, pancarditis	
Eyes		Conjunctivitis, iritis,‡ choroiditis,‡ retinal hemorrhage or detachment,‡ panophthalmitis‡	Keratitis
Liver		Mild or recurrent hepatitis	
Respiratory system		Nonexudative sore throat, nonproductive cough, adult respiratory distress syndrome‡	
Kidneys		Microscopic hematuria or proteinuria	
Genitourinary system		Orchitis‡	
Constitutional symptoms	Minor	Severe malaise and fatigue	Fatigue

From Steere AC: *N Engl J Med* 321:586, 1989.

*Classification by stages provides a guideline for the illness's manifestations, but timing and sequence can vary greatly.

†Systems are listed from the most to the least commonly affected.

‡Inclusion of this manifestation is based on one or a few cases.

Etiological agents, factors, and diseases associated with aseptic meningitis

Viruses

Enteroviruses (echoviruses, coxsackieviruses A and B, polioviruses, and enteroviruses)

Arboviruses (in the United States: Eastern equine, Western equine, Venezuelan equine, St. Louis, Powassan, California and Colorado tick fever; in other areas of the world, many other arboviruses are important)

Mumps

Herpes simplex type 2

Human immunodeficiency

Adenoviruses

Varicella-zoster (VZ)

Epstein-Barr (EB)

Lymphocytic choriomeningitis

Encephalomyocarditis

Cytomegalovirus

Rhinoviruses

Measles

Rubella

Influenza A and B

Parainfluenza

Rotaviruses

Coronaviruses

Variola

Postvaccine reaction

Measles

Vaccinia

Polio

Rabies

Bacteria

Mycobacterium tuberculosis

Pyogenic—partially treated

Leptospira spp. (leptospirosis)

Treponema pallidum (syphilis)

Borrelia spp. (relapsing fever)

Borrelia burgdorferi (Lyme disease)

Nocardia spp. (nocardiosis)

Fungi

Blastomyces dermatitidis

Coccidioides immitis

Cryptococcus neoformans

Histoplasma capsulatum

Candida spp.

Other: *Alternaria* spp., *Aspergillus* spp., *Cephalosporium* spp., *Cladosporium trichoides*, *Dreschslera hawaiiensis*, *Paracoccidioides brasiliensis*, *Petriellidium boydii*, *Sporotrichum schenckii*, *Ustilago* spp., *Zygomycete* spp.

Rickettsia

R. rickettsii (Rocky Mountain spotted fever)

R. prowazekii (typhus)

Mycoplasma

M. pneumoniae

M. hominis

Parasites

Angiostrongylus cantonensis (eosinophilic meningitis)

Trichinella spiralis (trichinosis)

Toxoplasma gondii (toxoplasmosis)

Parameningeal infections
Malignancy

Leukemia

CNS tumor

Immune diseases

Behçet syndrome

Lupus erythematosus

Sarcoidosis

Miscellaneous

Kawasaki disease

Toxic shock syndrome

Heavy metal poisoning

Intrathecal injections (e.g., contrast media antibiotics)

Foreign bodies (shunt, reservoir)

Antimicrobial agents

Modified from Cherry JD: Aseptic meningitis and viral meningitis. In Feigen RD, Cherry JD, editors: *Textbook of pediatric infectious disease*, ed 2, Philadelphia, 1987, WB Saunders.

See *Primary Pediatric Care*, ed 3, p. 1424.

Characteristic cerebrospinal fluid findings in patients with meningitis

CSF findings	Bacterial	Viral	Fungal and tuberculous
Leukocytes			
Usual	>500	<500	<500
Range	0-200,000	0-2000	
Percent polymorphonuclear neutrophils			
Usual	>80%	<50%	<50%
Range	20%-100%	0-100%	
Glucose			
Usual	<40 mg/dl	>40 mg/dl	<40 mg/dl
Range	0-normal	30 mg/dl-normal	
Percent CSF/blood	<30	>50	
Protein			
Usual	>100 mg/dl	<100 mg/dl	>100 mg/dl
Range	Normal-1500 mg/dl	Normal-200 mg/dl	
Stains	Gram stain	—	India ink/acid-fast

See *Primary Pediatric Care,* ed 3, p. 1423.

Official levels of mental retardation and some developmental characteristics*

Level and title	IQ range	Estimated percentage of total retarded	Adaptive and developmental characteristics			
			Preschool age 0-5 (maturation and development)	School age 6-20 (training and education)	Adult ≥ 21 (social and vocational adequacy)
1. Profound	<20		Gross retardation; minimum capacity for functioning in sensorimotor areas; may need nursing care	Some motor development present; may respond to minimum or limited training in self-help	Some motor and speech development; may achieve very limited self-care; may need nursing care
2. Severe	20-35	5	Poor motor development; minimal speech; able to profit from training in self-help; little or no expressive skills	Can talk or learn to communicate; can be trained in elemental health habits; can profit from systematic habit training	May contribute partially to self-maintenance under complete supervision; can develop self-protection skills to a minimum useful level in controlled environment
3. Moderate	36-51	20	Can talk or learn to communicate; poor social awareness; fair motor development; profits from training in self-help; can be managed with moderate supervision	Can profit from training in social and occupational skills; unlikely to progress beyond second-grade level in academic subjects; may learn to travel alone in familiar places	May achieve self-maintenance in unskilled or semiskilled work under sheltered conditions; needs supervision and guidance when under mild social or economic stress
4. Mild	52-68	75	Can develop social and communication skills; minimal retardation in sensorimotor areas; often not distinguished from normal until later age	Can learn academic skills up to approximately sixth-grade level by late teens; can be guided toward social conformity; "educable"	Can usually achieve social and vocational skills adequate to minimum self-support but may need guidance and assistance when under unusual social or economic stress

*Definition of mental retardation: "Significantly subaverage general intellectual functioning existing concurrently with deficits in adaptive behavior and manifest during the developmental period."

See *Primary Pediatric Care*, ed 3, p. 409.

Microhematuria

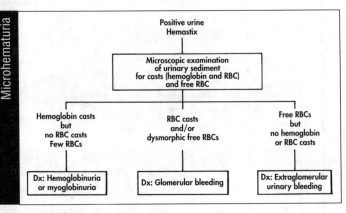

A clinical algorithm for microhematuria in children.
See *Primary Pediatric Care,* ed 3, p. 997.

Abnormalities of metabolism associated with unusual odor

Disease	Description of odor	Clinical features	Metabolic defect
Phenylketonuria	Musty, like a mouse, horse, wolf, or barn	Vomiting, progressive mental retardation and microcephaly, eczema, decreasing pigmentation, seizures, spasticity	Phenylalanine hydroxylase
Maple syrup urine disease	Maple syrup, burnt sugar, malt, caramel	Feeding difficulty, irregular respiration beginning in first week, marked acidosis, seizures, coma leading to death in first 1-2 years of life	Branched chain decarboxylase
		Intermittent form without mental retardation but with episodes of ataxia and lethargy that may progress to coma	
		Other variants, including thiamine, respond to treatment	
Oasthouse urine disease (methionine malabsorption syndrome)	Yeast, dried celery, malt, hops, beer	Diarrhea, mental retardation, spasticity, attacks of hyperpnea, fever, edema	Kidney and intestinal transport of methionine, branched chain amino acids, tyrosine, and phenylalanine
Odor of sweaty feet syndrome 1 (isovalericacidemia)	Sweaty feet, cheese	Recurrent bouts of acidosis, vomiting, dehydration, coma, mild to moderate mental retardation, aversion to protein foods	Isovaleryl CoA dehydrogenase

Continued.

See *Primary Pediatric Care*, ed 3, p. 1066.

Odor, metabolic causes

Abnormalities of metabolism associated with unusual odor—cont'd

Disease	Description of odor	Clinical features	Metabolic defect
Odor of sweaty feet syndrome 2 (*N*-butyric and *N*-hexanoic acidemia; may be same as odor of sweaty feet syndrome 1)	Sweaty feet	Poor feeding, weakness and lethargy developing in first week of life with acidosis, dehydration, seizures, and death in early months of life from bone marrow depression	Green acyldehydrogenase
Odor of cat urine syndrome (beta-methylcrotonylglycinuria)	Cat urine	Neurological symptoms resembling Werdnig-Hoffmann disease, failure to thrive, ketoacidosis Biotin-responsive form	Multiple carboxylase deficiency
Fish odor syndrome 1	Dead fish	Stigmata of Turner syndrome, neutropenia, recurrent infections, anemia, splenomegaly	Unknown
Fish odor syndrome 2 (tri-methylaminuria)	Dead or rotting fish, rancid butter, boiled cabbage	Normal development; has been induced in two premature infants by oral choline	Trimethylamine oxidase
Rancid butter syndrome	Rancid butter, boiled cabbage, decaying fish	Poor feeding, irritability, progressive neurological deterioration with coma and seizures, death caused by infection in first 3 months	Unknown; hypermethioninemia, hypertyrosinemia, and generalized aminoaciduria present; may be a form of acute tyrosinosis

Modified from Mace JW et al: *Clin Pediatr* 15:57, 1976; Hayden GF: *Postgrad Med* 67:110, 1980.

Criteria for oppositional defiant disorder*

A. A pattern of negativistic, hostile, and defiant behavior lasting at least 6 months, during which four (or more) of the following are present:
   1. Often loses temper
   2. Often argues with adults
   3. Often defies or refuses to comply with adults' requests or rules
   4. Often annoys people deliberately
   5. Often blames others for his or her own mistakes or misbehavior
   6. Often is touchy or easily annoyed by others
   7. Often is angry and resentful
   8. Often is spiteful or vindictive

   Note: A criterion is considered met only if the behavior occurs more often than is typically observed in individuals of comparable age and developmental level.

B. The disturbance in behavior causes clinically significant impairment in social, academic, or occupational functioning.

C. The behaviors do not occur exclusively during the course of a psychotic or mood disorder.

D. Criteria are not met for conduct disorder and, if the individual is 18 years of age or older, criteria are not met for antisocial personality disorder.

*From The American Psychiatric Association: *Diagnostic and statistical manual of mental disorders,* ed 4, Washington, DC, 1994, The Association.

Oppositional defiant disorder

See *Primary Pediatric Care,* ed 3, p. 671.

Classification of orbital cellulitis

Stage	Description
I Inflammatory edema	Inflammatory edema beginning in medial or lateral upper eyelid; usually nontender with only minimal skin changes. No induration, visual impairment, or limitation of extraocular movements.
II Orbital cellulitis	Edema of orbital contents with varying degrees of proptosis, chemosis, limitation of extraocular movement, and visual loss.
III Subperiosteal abscess	Proptosis down and out with signs of orbital cellulitis (usually severe). Abscess beneath the periosteum of the ethmoid, frontal, or maxillary bone (in that order of frequency).
IV Orbital abscess	Abscess within the fat or muscle cone in the posterior orbit. Severe chemosis and proptosis; complete ophthalmoplegia and moderate to severe visual loss present (globe displaced forward or down and out).
V Cavernous sinus thrombosis	Proptosis, globe fixation, severe loss of visual acuity, prostration, signs of meningitis; progresses to proptosis, chemosis, and visual loss in contralateral eye.

From Wald ER et al: *Pediatr Clin North Am* 28:787, 1981; modified from Chandler JR, Langenbrunner DJ, Stevens ER: *Laryngoscope* 80:1414, 1970.

See *Primary Pediatric Care,* ed 3, p. 1595.

Evaluation of petechiae and purpura

1. History and physical examination
Duration/speed of onset
"Sick versus well"
Distribution of lesions

2. Low platelet count (<150,000)
a. Blood smear
Verify low platelet count
Look for *microangiopathic changes*
  Kasabach-Merritt syndrome
  DIC/purpura fulminans
  Hemolytic uremic syndrome (HUS)
  Thrombotic thrombocytopenic purpura (TTP)
  Liver disease

b. PT, aPTT (±FDP, fibrinogen)
Abnormal

As above plus:
  Histiocytosis X
  Familial erythrophagocytic lymphohistiocytosis (FEL)

Normal
See below

c. Bone marrow examination
Decreased megakaryocytes

Aplasia, congenital
  Thrombocytopenia with absent radii (TAR) syndrome
  Fanconi anemia
  Bernard-Soulier syndrome
  Wiskott-Aldrich syndrome
  Metabolic disorders
Aplasia, acquired
  Idiopathic
  Nutritional (iron, vitamin B_{12}, folate)
  Drug, chemical, toxin, radiation
  Rubella, other "TORCH"
Infiltration
  Leukemia, lymphoma
  Neuroblastoma or other
    metastatic solid tumor
  Storage disease

See *Primary Pediatric Care*, ed 3, p. 1069.

Continued

Evaluation of petechiae and purpura—cont'd

Normal or increased megakaryocytes

Immune destruction

  Immune thrombocytopenic purpura (ITP) (acute and chronic)
  Alloimmune thrombocytopenia
  Posttransfusion purpura
  Drugs
  HIV/AIDS

Other

  Histiocytosis X
  Virally associated hematophagocytic syndrome (VAHS)
  FEL
  Intravascular prosthesis
  May-Hegglin anomaly
  Hypersplenism with sequestration

3. Normal platelet count (>150,000)
Platelet dysfunction, congenital

Glanzmann thrombasthenia
Bernard-Soulier syndrome
Wiskott-Aldrich syndrome
Storage pool defect

Platelet dysfunction, acquired

Aspirin or aspirin-like drugs
Liver disease
Uremia
Paraproteinemia (dysgammaglobulinemia, cystic fibrosis)

Von Willebrand disease
Vascular defect, congenital

Ehlers-Danlos syndrome
Osler-Weber-Rendu syndrome

Vascular defect, acquired

Trauma (lacerations, abuse)
Lacerations
Abuse
Factitious
Vasculitis
  Drugs
  Infection (bacterial, viral, rickettsial)
  Henoch-Schönlein purpura
Senile purpura
Steroid purpura
Scurvy

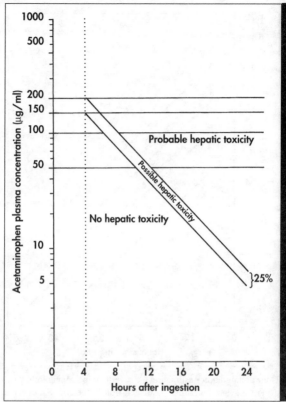

Rumack-Matthew nomogram for estimating the probability of hepatic toxicity after a single acute acetaminophen ingestion. The lower solid diagonol line is placed 25% below the upper solid diagonol line, which divides the "no hepatic toxicity" area. This allows for potential errors in estimating the time after ingestion of the acetaminophen and potential errors in the measurement of acetaminophen plasma levels. (Adapted from Rumack BH, Matthew H: *Pediatrics* 55:871, 1975.)
See *Primary Pediatric Care,* ed 3, p. 1742.

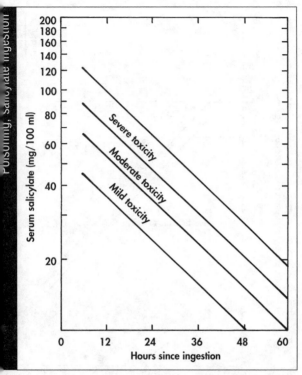

Done nomogram for estimating the severity of poisoning following a single acute salicylate ingestion. (Adapted from Done AK: Salicylate intoxication: significance of measurements of salicylate in blood in cases of acute ingestion, *Pediatrics* 26:800, 1960.)
See *Primary Pediatric Care,* ed 3, p. 1741.

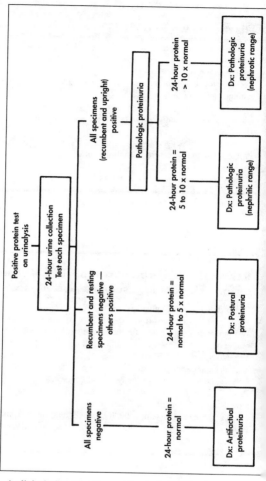

A clinical algorithm for proteinuria in children.
See *Primary Pediatric Care*, ed 3, p. 1078.

Diagnostic workup for ITP

Studies to be performed when a patient who has ITP does not fit all the criteria listed in the box to the left or if apparent AITPC does not resolve within 6 months:

Bone marrow examination
Immunoglobulin levels
Reticulocyte count
Direct and indirect antiglobulin (Coombs) test
Urinalysis
Antinuclear antibody levels
Prothrombin and partial thromboplastin times
Bleeding time
Human immunodeficiency virus antibody

See *Primary Pediatric Care,* ed 3, p. 1367.

Recommended procedures for the collection of forensic data in case of suspected rape

Combed and plucked pubic hair
Wet mount of secretions from the vaginal vault
Wet mount and fixed smear for the detection of both motile and dead sperm
Vaginal aspirate for acid phosphatase
Vaginal aspirate for p30 and MH-5 testing
Cervical cultures for both chlamydia and gonorrhea
Rectal cultures for gonorrhea even if sodomy has not occurred
Oral culture for gonorrhea if fellatio occurred
Dried secretions from skin, pubic hair, or clothing for analysis
Blood tests: ABO typing, syphilis, pregnancy test, and HIV test (if patient requests it)

See *Primary Pediatric Care,* ed 3, p. 1754.

Staging of Reye syndrome

	I	II	III	IV	V
Level of consciousness	Lethargy; follows verbal commands	Combative/stupor; verbalizes inappropriately	Coma	Coma	Coma
Posture	Normal	Normal	Decorticate	Decerebrate	Flaccid
Response to pain	Purposeful	Purposeful/nonpurposeful	Decorticate	Decerebrate	None
Pupillary reaction	Brisk	Sluggish	Sluggish	Sluggish	None
Oculocephalic reflex (doll's eyes)	Normal	Conjugate deviation	Conjugate deviation	Inconsistent or absent	None

From National Institutes of Health Consensus Development Conference: *JAMA* 246:2442, 1981.

See *Primary Pediatric Care*, ed 3, p. 1544.

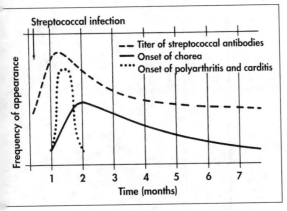

Onset of rheumatic manifestations in relationship to antecedent streptococcal infection and ASO titer. (Modified from Stollerman GH: *Rheumatic fever and streptococcal infection,* New York, 1975, Grune & Stratton.)

See *Primary Pediatric Care,* ed 3, p. 1549.

Salpingitis: clinical criteria for diagnosis

Minimum criteria

Empirical treatment of PID should be instituted on the basis of the presence of all of the following three minimum clinical criteria for pelvic inflammation and in the absence of an established cause other than PID:

- Lower abdominal tenderness
- Adnexal tenderness
- Cervical motion tenderness

Additional criteria

For women who have severe clinical signs, more elaborate diagnostic evaluation is warranted because incorrect diagnosis and management may cause unnecessary morbidity. These additional criteria may be used to increase the specificity of the diagnosis.

Listed below are the *routine* criteria for diagnosing PID:

- Oral temperature >38.3° C
- Abnormal cervical or vaginal discharge
- Elevated erythrocyte sedimentation rate
- Elevated C-reactive protein
- Laboratory documentation of cervical infection with *N. gonorrhoeae* or *C. trachomatis*

From Centers for Disease Control and Prevention: *MMWR* 42(no RR-14):77, 1993.

See *Primary Pediatric Care,* ed 3, p. 1590.

Role of the history in the evaluation of school learning problems

Aspect	Findings suggesting specific learning disabilities
School functioning	
Academic achievement	Discrete delays in select subjects (e.g., language); adequate early performance with difficulties emerging later (e.g., mathematics, writing)
Classroom behavior	Long-standing, pervasive problems with inattention, impulsivity, overactivity; disorganization and poor strategy formation; depression, moodiness
Attendance	Excessive absenteeism; school avoidance
Past psychoeducational testing	Discrepancy between cognitive abilities and academic achievement
Special required school services	Response to "diagnostic teaching"
Perinatal history	"Clusters" of adverse events; maternal alcohol or drug intake
Medical history	Recurrent and/or persistent otitis media; iron deficiency anemia; lead poisoning; seizures; frequent accidents; chronic use of medication
Development	Delayed or disordered language acquisition and communication skills; subtle delays in select milestones; "uneven" pattern of skills and interests
Behavioral history	Long-standing, pervasive problems with attention span, impulsivity, overactivity; sadness; acting out; poor self-esteem
Family history	Learning problems, school failure among first-degree relatives
Social history	Child abuse or neglect; other stressors

See *Primary Pediatric Care*, ed 3, p. 691.

Role of the physical examination in evaluation of school learning problems

Aspect	Findings suggesting specific learning disabilities
General observations	Sadness, anxiety, short attention span, impulsivity, overactivity; tics
Phenotypical features	Stigmata of genetic syndromes (e.g., sex chromosome abnormalities, fetal alcohol syndrome); minor congenital anomalies
Skin	Multiple café-au-lait spots; "ash leaf" spots, adenoma sebaceum
Tympanic membranes	Signs of recurrent or chronic otitis media
Genitalia	Delayed sexual maturation in boys
Growth measurements	Short stature; microcephaly and macrocephaly
Sensory screening	Poor hearing or vision

See *Primary Pediatric Care,* ed 3, p. 692.

Symptoms and signs associated with shock

Tachycardia

Hypotension

Oliguria

Capillary refill >3 seconds

Tachypnea

Dry mucous membranes

Altered mental status

From Crone RK: *Pediatr Clin North Am* 27:525, 1980.

See *Primary Pediatric Care,* ed 3, p. 1765.

Summary of clinical and laboratory data associated with staphylococcal TSS

Condition	Relative frequency of occurrence (%)
Clinical	
Fever	100
Temperature >40° C (>104° F)	70
Rash	100
Diffuse erythema	87
Desquamation	90
Myalgia	99
Hypotension (orthostatic hypotension or syncope)	95
Disorientation, irritability, or lethargy	89
Diarrhea	83
Vomiting	82
Sore throat	80
Strawberry tongue	80
Headache	78
Abdominal pain and tenderness	70
Vaginal hyperemia	67
Conjunctivitis	65
Vaginal discharge	42
Stiff neck	36
Arthralgia	15
Joint effusion	12
Adult respiratory distress syndrome	10
Laboratory	
Hematological	
Increased fibrinolytic split products	100
Immature neutrophils	95
Anemia	82
Leukocytosis	76
Prolonged prothrombin time	70
Decreased fibrinogen	68
Thrombocytopenia	64
Prolonged partial thromboplastin time	60
Metabolic	
Hypoproteinemia	95
Hypoalbuminemia	85
Hypocalcemia	83
Hypokalemia	75
Hypophosphatemia	62
Hyponatremia	47
Hepatic	
Elevated hepatic enzymes	67
Hyperbilirubinemia	63

See *Primary Pediatric Care*, ed 3, p. 1614. *Continued*

Summary of clinical and laboratory data associated with
staphylococcal TSS—cont'd

Condition	Relative frequency of occurrence (%)
Renal	
Pyuria	100
Increased creatinine	82
Increased BUN	75
Proteinuria	70
Microscopic hematuria	50
Musculoskeletal	
Increased creatinine phosphokinase	75
Metabolic acidosis	75
Myoglobinuria	66

Case definition of staphylococcal toxic shock syndrome

Fever: temperature >38.9° C

Rash: diffuse macular erythroderma; desquamation of palms and
soles 1 to 2 weeks after onset of illness

Hypotension: systolic blood pressure 90 mm Hg for adults or below
5th percentile by age for children under 16 years of age; orthostatic drop in diastolic blood pressure 15 mm Hg from lying to
sitting, or orthostatic syncope

Multisystem involvement—three or more of the following:
Gastrointestinal: vomiting or diarrhea at onset of illness
Muscular: severe myalgia or creatinine phosphokinase level at least
twice the upper limit of normal for laboratory
Mucous membrane: vaginal, oropharyngeal, or conjunctival hypere-
mia
Renal: blood urea nitrogen (BUN) or creatinine at least twice the
upper limit of normal for laboratory or urinary sediment with
pyuria (>5 white cells per high-power field) in the absence of
urinary tract infection
Hepatic: total bilirubin, serum glutamic-oxalo-acetic transaminase
(SGOT), or serum glutamic-pyruvate transaminase (SGPT) at
least twice the upper limit of normal for laboratory
Hematological: platelets <100,000/mm³
CNS: disorientation or alterations in consciousness without focal
neurological signs when fever and hypotension are absent

Negative results on the following tests, if obtained:
Blood, throat, cerebrospinal fluid (CSF) cultures
Rise in antibody titer: Rocky Mountain spotted fever, leptospirosis,
and rubeola

See _Primary Pediatric Care,_ ed 3, p. 1616.

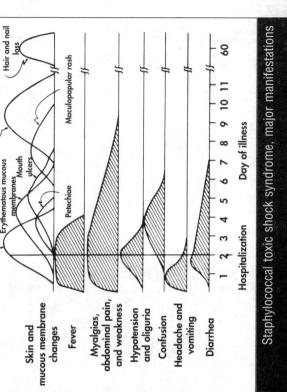

Staphylococcal toxic shock syndrome, major manifestations

Major systemic, skin, and mucous membrane manifestations of toxic shock syndrome. (From Chesney PJ et al: *JAMA* 246:743, 1981.)
See *Primary Pediatric Care,* ed 3, p. 1613.

Indications for sweat testing

Respiratory	Gastrointestinal	Other
Lower respiratory	**Neonatal**	Aspermia
Chronic cough	Meconium ileus	Absent vas deferens
Recurrent/chronic pneumonia	Meconium plug	Metabolic alkalosis
Recurrent wheezing	Intestinal atresia	Salty taste
Atelectasis	Prolonged jaundice	Salt crystals
Bronchiectasis	Malabsorption	Positive family history
Clubbing	Steatorrhea	Hypoprothrombinemia
Colonization with mucoid PA	Edema and hypoproteinemia	
Hemoptysis	Failure to thrive	
Pneumothorax	Rectal prolapse	
Upper respiratory	Recurrent intussusception	
Nasal polyps	Recurrent pancreatitis	
Pansinusitis	Recurrent ABD obstruction	
	Cirrhosis	
	Cholecystitis	

See *Primary Pediatric Care*, ed 3, p. 418.

Surveillance case definition for congenital syphilis

For reporting purposes, congenital syphilis includes cases of congenitally acquired syphilis in infants and children, as well as syphilitic stillbirths.

A CONFIRMED CASE of congenital syphilis is an infant in whom *Treponema pallidum* is identified by darkfield microscopy, fluorescent antibody, or other specific stains in specimens from lesions, placenta, umbilical cord, or autopsy material.

A PRESUMPTIVE CASE of congenital syphilis is either of the following:

A. Any infant whose mother had untreated or inadequately treated* syphilis at delivery, regardless of findings in the infant

OR

B. Any infant or child who has a reactive treponemal test for syphilis and any one of the following:
1. Any evidence of congenital syphilis on physical examination† or
2. Any evidence of congenital syphilis on long-bone radiograph or
3. Reactive cerebrospinal fluid VDRL‡ or
4. Elevated CSF cell count or protein (without other cause)‡ or
5. Quantitative nontreponemal serological titers that are fourfold higher than the mother's (both drawn at birth) or
6. Reactive test for FTA-ABS-19S-IgM antibody‡

A SYPHILITIC STILLBIRTH is defined as a fetal death in which the mother had untreated or inadequately treated syphilis at delivery of a fetus after a 20-week gestation or of a fetus weighing more than 500 g.

From Congenital syphilis—New York City, 1986-1988, *MMWR* 38:825, 1989.

*Inadequate treatment consists of any nonpenicillin therapy or penicillin given less than 30 days before delivery.

†Signs in an infant (under 2 years of age) may include hepatosplenomegaly, characteristic skin rash, condyloma lata, snuffles, jaundice (syphilitic hepatitis), pseudoparalysis, or edema (nephrotic syndrome). Stigmata in an older child may include interstitial keratitis, nerve deafness, anterior bowing of shins, frontal bossing, mulberry molars, Hutchinson's teeth, saddle nose, rhagades, or Clutton joints.

‡Distinguishing between congenital and acquired syphilis may be difficult in a seropositive child after infancy. Signs may not be obvious and stigmata may not yet have developed. Abnormal values for CSF VDRL, cell count, and protein, as well as IgM antibodies, may be found in either congenital or acquired syphilis. Findings on long-bone radiographs may help because these would indicate congenital syphilis. The decision may ultimately be based on maternal history and clinical judgment; the possibility of sexual abuse also needs to be considered.

See *Primary Pediatric Care,* ed 3, p. 1589.

Criteria for the diagnosis of acute idiopathic thrombocytopenia of childhood

Platelet count ≤20,000
Normal complete blood count, including the absolute neutrophil count and the examination of red blood cells, white blood cells, and platelet morphology on the blood smear
Age 1 to 9 years
Otherwise patient well
Acute onset (symptomatic <2 weeks)
Preceding viral illness within 1 to 3 weeks
Normal size spleen
No personal history or family history of other possible autoimmune disorders (e.g., hemolytic anemia, nephritis, thyroiditis, collagen-vascular disease, or frequent infections)

See *Primary Pediatric Care,* ed 3, p. 1366.

Primary brain tumors of childhood

Supratentorial (cerebral hemisphere)

Astrocytoma
Oligodendroglioma
Ependymoma
Choroid plexus papilloma
Meningioma

Midline (diencephalon)

Craniopharyngioma
Pinealoma
Optic nerve glioma

Infratentorial (brainstem and cerebellum)

Astrocytoma (cerebellum)
Medulloblastoma (cerebellum)
Glioma (brainstem)
Ependymoma

Other

Primitive neuroectodermal tumors

See *Primary Pediatric Care,* ed 3, p. 1209.

Therapeutic Modalities

Amebiasis
Anesthetics, local and regional
Antidotes
Antimicrobial prophylaxis, clinical situations
Antimicrobial prophylaxis, specific pathogens
Apnea, newborn
Arthritis, juvenile
Asthma
Asystole and pulseless arrest
Bradycardia
Cephalosporins
Dehydration
Diarrhea, acute
Diarrheal solutions
Disseminated intravascular coagulation
Encopresis, nonretentive
Encopresis, retentive
Endocarditis, infection prophylaxis
Fever without source, child
Fever without source, infant
Gastrointestinal hemorrhage
Heart failure
High blood pressure
HIV-seropositive mothers' infants
Hyperkalemia
Hypothyroidism
Infections, selected
Lead poisoning
Leukemia
Lyme disease
Otitis media, acute
Rabies, postexposure
Rabies vaccination
Staphylococcal toxic shock syndrome
Status epilepticus

Treatment of amebiasis

Severity of disease	Drugs	Administration	Total daily dose
Asymptomatic carrier (cyst passer) and mild intraluminal disease	Iodoquinol OR	3×/day for 20 days (PO)	40 mg/kg/day (max: 2 g)
	Diloxanide furoate OR	3×/day for 10 days (PO)	20-30 mg/kg/day (max: 1500 g)
	Paromomycin	3×/day for 7 days (PO)	30 mg/kg/day (max: 1500 g)
Moderate to severe intestinal disease (dysentery)	Metronidazole (followed by one of the three drugs listed above for asymptomatic carriers)	3×/day for 10 days (PO)	35-50 mg/kg/day
Extraintestinal amebiasis or ameboma	Metronidazole (followed by one of the three drugs listed above for asymptomatic carriers) OR	3×/day for 10 days (PO)	35-50 mg/kg/day
	Dehydroemetine PLUS	2×/day for 10 days (IM)	1-1.5 mg/kg/day (max: 90 mg)
	Chloroquine	2×/day for 21 days (PO)	10 mg base/kg/day (max: 300 mg base)

See *Primary Pediatric Care,* ed 3, p. 1480.

Suggested maximal doses of local anesthetics (mg/kg)*

Drug (concentration)†	Caudal/lumbar epidural	Peripheral‡	Subcutaneous‡
Esters			
Chloroprocaine (1.0% infiltration) (2%-3% epidural)	8-10§	8-10§	8-10§
Procaine	NR	8-10§	8-10§
Amides			
Lidocaine (0.5%-2.0%) (0.5%-1.0% infiltration) (1%-2% peripheral, epidural, subcutaneous) (5% spinal)	5-7§	5-7§	5-7§
Bupivacaine (0.0625%-0.5%) (0.125%-0.25%)	2-3§	2-3§	2-3§
Prilocaine (0.5%-1% infiltration) (1%-1.5% peripheral) (2%-3% epidural)	5-7§‖	5-7§‖	5-7§‖

*These are suggested safe upper limits; direct intraarterial or intravenous injection of even a fraction of these doses may result in systemic toxicity or death.
†Concentrations are in mg percent; e.g., a 1% solution contains 10 mg/ml.
‡Epinephrine should never be added to local anesthetic solution administered in area of an end artery (e.g., penile nerve block).
§The higher dose is recommended only with the concomitant use of epinephrine 1:200,000.
‖Total adult dose should not exceed 600 mg. Should be used with caution in neonates.
NR, Not recommended.

See *Primary Pediatric Care*, ed 3, p. 313.

Common antidotes

Drug	Diagnostic findings requiring treatment	Antidote	Dosage
Acetaminophen	History of ingestion and toxic serum level	N-acetylcysteine	140 mg/kg/dose PO, then 70 mg/kg/dose q 4 hr PO × 17
Anticholinergics Antihistamines Atropine Phenothiazines Tricyclic antidepressants	Supraventricular tachycardia (hemodynamic compromise) Unresponsive ventricular dysrhythmia, seizures, pronounced hallucinations or agitation	Physostigmine	Child: 0.5 mg IV slowly (over 3 min) q 10 min prn (maximum: 2 mg) Adult: 1-2 mg IV slowly q 10 min prn (maximum: 4 mg in 30 min)
Cholinergics	Cholinergic crisis: salivation, lacrimation, urination, defecation, convulsions, fasciculations	Atropine sulfate Physostigmine Insecticides	0.05 mg/kg/dose (usual dose 1-5 mg; test dose for child 0.01 mg/kg) q 4-6 hr IV or more frequently prn
Carbon monoxide	Headache, seizure, coma, dysrhythmias	Oxygen, hyperbaric oxygen	100% oxygen (half-life 40 min); consider hyperbaric chamber
Cyanide	Cyanosis, seizures, cardiopulmonary arrest, coma	Amyl nitrite Sodium nitrite (3%) Sodium thiosulfate (25%) Also consider hyperbaric oxygen	Inhale pearl q 60-120 sec 0.27 ml (8.7 mg)/kg (adult: 10 ml [300 mg]) IV slowly (Hb ≥10 g/dl) 1.35 mL (325 mg)/kg (adult: 12.5 g) IV slowly (Hb ≥10 g/dl)
Ethylene glycol	Metabolic acidosis, urine Ca^{++} oxalate crystals	Ethanol (100% absolute, 1 ml-790 mg)	1 ml/kg in D5W IV over 15 min, then 0.16 ml (125 mg)/kg/hr IV; maintain ethanol level of 100 mg/dl

See *Primary Pediatric Care*, ed 3, p. 1687.

Iron	Hypotension, shock, coma, serum iron >350 mg/dl (or greater than iron-binding capacity)	Deferoxamine	Shock or coma: 15 mg/kg/hr IV for 8 hr; if no shock or coma 90 mg/kg/dose IM q 8 hr
Phenothiazines Chlorpromazine Thioridazine	Extrapyramidal dyskinesis, oculogyric crisis	Diphenhydramine (Benadryl)	1-2 mg/kg/dose (maximum: 50 mg/dose) q 6 hr IV, PO
Methanol	Metabolic acidosis, blurred vision; level >20 mg/dl	Ethanol (100% absolute)	1 ml/kg in D5W over 15 min, then 0.16 ml (125 mg)/kg/hr IV
Methemoglobin Nitrate Nitrites Sulfonamide	Cyanosis, methemoglobin level >30%, dyspnea	Methylene blue (1% solution)	1-2 mg (0.1-0.2 ml)/kg/dose IV; repeat in 4 hr if necessary
Narcotics Heroin Codeine Propoxyphene	Respiratory depression, hypotension, coma	Naloxone (Narcan)	0.1 mg/kg up to 0.8 mg initially IV; if no response give 2 mg IV
Organophosphates Malathion Parathion	Cholinergic crisis: salivation, lacrimation, urination, defecation, convulsions, fasciculations	Atropine sulfate	0.05 mg/kg/dose (usual dose 1-5 mg; test dose for child 0.01 mg/kg) q 4-6 hr IV or more frequently prn
		Pralidoxime	After atropine, 20-50 mg/kg/dose (maximum: 2000 mg) IV slowly (<50 mg/min) q 8 hr IV prn × 3

From Barkin RM: Toxicologic emergencies, *Pediatr Ann* 19:632, 1990.

Clinical situations in which prophylaxis with antimicrobial agents has proved effective

Body site	Infection to be prevented	Agents	Recommended dosage
Conjunctivae	Neonatal gonococcal ophthalmia	1% silver nitrate, 0.5% erythromycin, 1% tetracycline, penicillin	Applied topically once shortly after delivery
Abnormal heart valve	Bacterial endocarditis (e.g., after dental extraction)	Penicillin, ampicillin	*Standard-risk patients, oral procedures:* penicillin V, 2 g PO, then 1 g 6 hours later; *high-risk patients, dental, or all patients, GU or GI tract procedures:* ampicillin, 2 g IM or IV plus gentamicin, 1.5-2 mg/kg 30 min before and 8 hours after procedure See Kaiser AB: *N Engl J Med* 315:1129, 1986.
Surgical wound	Serious postoperative wound infection	Appropriate for expected contaminants	
Middle ear	Recurrent otitis media	Amoxicillin, sulfisoxazole	5-10 mg/kg given q12h 40-50 mg/kg given q12h (given during winter and spring)
Urinary tract	Recurrent infection	Trimethoprim/sulfamethoxazole, nitrofurantoin	2 mg TMP and 10 mg SMX/kg once daily 1-2 mg/kg once daily Duration: months to years, depending on clinical situation
Human/animal bite wound*	Wound infection, cellulitis	Amoxicillin/clavulanate	40 mg of the amoxicillin component/kg/day given q8h for 5-7 days

Modified from Peter G et al, editors: Report of the Committee on Infectious Diseases: *1994 Red Book*, ed 23, Elk Grove Village, Ill, 1994, The American Academy of Pediatrics.
*Efficacy of treatment has not been established.

See *Primary Pediatric Care*, ed 3, p. 392.

Antimicrobial prophylaxis against specific pathogens

Pathogen	Disease to be prevented	Antimicrobial agent	Dose	Duration of therapy
Bacteria				
Bordetella pertussis	Secondary cases of pertussis in household contacts	Erythromycin estolate	40-50 mg/kg/day in 4 doses (not to exceed 2 g/day)	14 days
Chlamydia trachomatis*	Urogenital infections in exposed individuals	Doxycycline (>8 yr) **or** azithromycin (adolescents) **or** erythromycin	200 mg/day in 2 doses 1 g	7 days 1 dose PO
			40-50 mg/kg/day in 4 doses (not to exceed 2 g/day)	7 days
Corynebacterium diphtheriae*	Diphtheria in unimmunized contacts	Benzathine, penicillin **or** erythromycin	*<30 kg:* 600,00 U *>30 kg:* 1.2 million U 40-50 mg/kg/day in 4 doses (not to exceed 2 g/day)	1 dose IM 7 days
Haemophilus influenzae	Secondary cases of systemic infection in close contacts <1 yr of age and in children 12-47 mo who are not fully immunized	Rifampin	*≤1 mo:* 10-20 mg/kg *>1 mo:* 20 mg/kg (maximum 600 mg)	Once a day for 4 days
Mycobacterium tuberculosis	Overt pulmonary or metastatic infection	Isoniazid	10-20 mg/kg (not to exceed 300 mg)	Once a day for 9 days

Modified from Peter G et al, editors: *Report of the Committee on Infectious Diseases: 1994 Red Book*, ed 23, Elk Grove Village, Ill, 1994, The American Academy of Pediatrics.

*Efficacy of treatment has not been established.

Continued.

See *Primary Pediatric Care*, ed 3, p. 392.

Antimicrobial prophylaxis against specific pathogens—cont'd

Pathogen	Disease to be prevented	Antimicrobial agent	Dose	Duration of therapy
Bacteria—cont'd				
Neisseria meningitidis	Meningococcemia in exposed susceptible individuals	Rifampin	≤1 mo: 5-10 mg/kg >1 mo: 10 mg/kg (maximum 600 mg)	q12h for 4 doses
Neisseria gonorrhoeae	Gonococcal infection in exposed individuals; ophthalmia neonatorum	Ceftriaxone **or** cefixime **or** zofloxicin (≥18 yr)	250 mg 400 or 800 mg 400 mg	1 dose IM 1 dose PO 1 dose PO
Streptococcus pneumoniae	Fulminant pneumococcal infection in individuals with asplenia or sickle cell disease	Penicillin V	125 mg	2 times/day for life
Group A streptococcus	Recurrent rheumatic fever	Benzathine penicillin **or** penicillin V **or** sulfadiazine	1.2 million U 125-250 mg <27 kg: 0.5 g >27 kg: 1 kg	Every 4 wk 2 times/day Once a day for life Once a day for life
Group B streptococcus	Neonatal infection	Ampicillin	Mother: 2 g IV given intrapartum, followed by 1 g q4h until delivery Infant: 50 mg/kg IM q12h for 2 days	
Treponema pallidum	Syphilis in exposed individuals	Benzathine penicillin	2.4 million U	1 dose IM

Organism	Indication	Drug	Dosage	Duration
*Vibrio cholerae**	Cholera in close contacts	Tetracycline or trimethoprim-sulfamethoxazole	250 mg q6h (>8 yr) 5 mg/kg as trimethoprim 2 times/day	3 days 3 days
*Yersinia pestis**	Plague in household contacts or individuals exposed to pneumonic disease	Tetracycline (>8 yr) or sulfonamide	15 mg/kg/day in 4 doses 40 mg/kg/day in 4 doses	7 days 7 days
Parasites				
Plasmodium species (malaria)	Overt infection in endemic areas	Chloroquine	5 mg/kg base once a week (maximum 300 mg base), beginning 2 wk before entering endemic area, while in area, and for 6 wk after leaving area	
Viruses				
Influenza A	Influenza in individuals at risk of complications	Amantadine	1-9 yr: 2-4.4 mg/kg q12h (maximum 150 mg/day) >9 yr: 100 mg q12h	Duration of influenza outbreak
Other				
Pneumocystis carinii	Pneumonia in a compromised host	Trimethoprim-sulfamethoxazole	5 mg trimethoprim/25 mg sulfamethoxazole	Once a day while patient is undergoing chemotherapy

Modified from Peter G et al, editors: Report of the Committee on Infectious Diseases: *1994 Red Book*, ed 23, Elk Grove Village, Ill, 1994, The American Academy of Pediatrics.
*Efficacy of treatment has not been established.

Treatment of apnea in newborns

Tactile stimulation. Gentle tapping on the infant's heel usually suffices. A pulsating waterbed sometimes is used for recurrent episodes.

Pharmacological intervention with methylxanthines (theophylline or caffeine). A loading dose of theophylline (5 mg/kg) is followed by maintenance at 1 to 2 mg/kg/dose (twice a day). Caffeine usually is given as 20 mg/kg loading dose orally, followed by 5 mg/kg/day.

Continuous positive airway pressure by nasal prongs.

Small increases in inspired oxygen from 21% to 25%, with monitoring of the response to maintain the arterial oxygen pressure (PaO_2) between 50 and 90 mm Hg.

Endotracheal intubation with positive end-expiratory pressure may be required for a short period in some cases.

See *Primary Pediatric Care*, ed 3, p. 538.

Medications for juvenile arthritis

Nonsteroidal antiinflammatory drugs (NSAIDs) currently approved by the FDA for use in children

Salicylates
Indomethacin
Tolmetin sodium
Naproxen
Ibuprofen

Nonsteroidal antiinflammatory drugs (NSAIDs) not yet approved by the FDA for use in children

Diclofenac sodium
Fenoprofen
Flurbiprofen
Ketoprofen
Phenylbutazone
Piroprofen
Piroxicam
Proquazone
Meclofenamate sodium
Sulindac

Slower-acting antirheumatic drugs (SAARDs)
Gold preparations

Gold sodium thiomalate
Aurothioglucose
Auranofin

Hydroxychloroquine

D-Penicillamine
Sulfasalazine
Methotrexate

Corticosteroids

Systemic
Intraarticular

Cytotoxic drugs

Azathioprine
Chlorambucil
Cyclophosphamide
Methotrexate

Other therapies

Pheresis
Intravenous immune globulin
Cyclosporin A

See *Primary Pediatric Care,* ed 3, p. 1384.

Arthritis, juvenile

Therapy for acute asthma

Drug	Mode	Dosage
Antiinflammatory		
Methylprednisolone	Intravenous	2 mg/kg load, then 2 mg/kg/day ÷ q 6 hr
Hydrocortisone	Intravenous	4-8 mg/kg load (max 250 mg), then 8 mg/kg/day ÷ q 6 hr
Beclomethasone dipropionate	Metered dose inhaler	1-2 puffs q 4-6 hrs
Cromolyn sodium	Nebulized (10 mg/ml)	20 mg q 6 hr
Nedocromil sodium	Metered dose inhaler	2 puffs q 6 hr
Adrenergic		
Epinephrine (1:1000)	Subcutaneous	0.01 ml/kg/dose (max 0.5 ml) q 15-20 min × 3
Sus-Phrine (1:200)	Subcutaneous	0.005 ml/kg/dose (max 0.15 ml) q 6 hr
Albuterol	Nebulized (5 mg/ml)	0.05-0.15 mg/kg q 1-3 hr (max 5 mg)
Intermittent		0.15-0.3 mg/kg q 1 hr continuously
Continuous		2-4 puffs q 1-3 hr
Metered dose inhaler		
Terbutaline	Nebulized (11 mg/ml)	0.1-0.3 mg/kg q 2-6 hr (max 11mg)
	Subcutaneous (0.5 mg/ml)	0.01 mg/kg q 20-30 min × 3 (max 0.25 mg)
	Intravenous	0.002 mg/kg load over 5 min, 0.0045 mg/kg/hr
Isoproterenol	Nebulized (5 mg/ml)	0.05-0.1 mg/kg q 2-6 hr (max 2.5 mg)
	Intravenous	0.05 μg/kg/min, then titrate by 0.05-0.1 μg/kg/min q15-30 min (max 1 μg/kg/min)
Theophylline	Intravenous (25 mg/ml)	6 mg/kg load, then <1 yr = 0.65 mg/kg/hr >1 yr = 0.9 mg/kg/hr; modify load if history of recent theophylline dosage, noting that 1 mg/kg = 2 μg/ml serum level
Anticholinergic		
Atropine	Nebulized	0.05 mg/kg
Glycopyrrolate	Nebulized (0.2 mg/ml)	0.4 mg q 4-6 hr
Ipratropium bromide	Nebulized	250-500 μg q 6 hr
	Metered dose inhaler	2-4 puffs q 4-6 hr

See *Primary Pediatric Care,* ed 3, p. 1771.

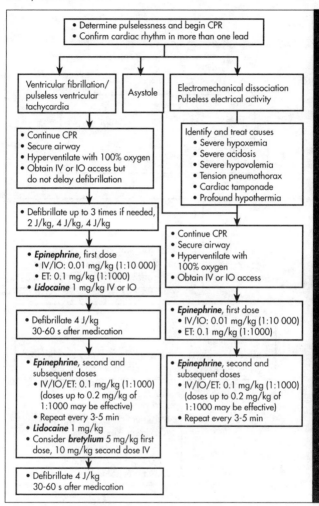

- Determine pulselessness and begin CPR
- Confirm cardiac rhythm in more than one lead

| Ventricular fibrillation/ pulseless ventricular tachycardia | Asystole | Electromechanical dissociation Pulseless electrical activity |

Ventricular fibrillation / pulseless ventricular tachycardia branch:

- Continue CPR
- Secure airway
- Hyperventilate with 100% oxygen
- Obtain IV or IO access but do not delay defibrillation

↓

- Defibrillate up to 3 times if needed, 2 J/kg, 4 J/kg, 4 J/kg

↓

- *Epinephrine*, first dose
  - IV/IO: 0.01 mg/kg (1:10 000)
  - ET: 0.1 mg/kg (1:1000)
- *Lidocaine* 1 mg/kg IV or IO

↓

- Defibrillate 4 J/kg 30-60 s after medication

↓

- *Epinephrine*, second and subsequent doses
  - IV/IO/ET: 0.1 mg/kg (1:1000) (doses up to 0.2 mg/kg of 1:1000 may be effective)
  - Repeat every 3-5 min
- *Lidocaine* 1 mg/kg
- Consider *bretylium* 5 mg/kg first dose, 10 mg/kg second dose IV

↓

- Defibrillate 4 J/kg 30-60 s after medication

Electromechanical dissociation / Pulseless electrical activity branch:

- Identify and treat causes
  - Severe hypoxemia
  - Severe acidosis
  - Severe hypovolemia
  - Tension pneumothorax
  - Cardiac tamponade
  - Profound hypothermia

↓

- Continue CPR
- Secure airway
- Hyperventilate with 100% oxygen
- Obtain IV or IO access

↓

- *Epinephrine*, first dose
  - IV/IO: 0.01 mg/kg (1:10 000)
  - ET: 0.1 mg/kg (1:1000)

↓

- *Epinephrine*, second and subsequent doses
  - IV/IO/ET: 0.1 mg/kg (1:1000) (doses up to 0.2 mg/kg of 1:1000 may be effective)
  - Repeat every 3-5 min

Asystole and pulseless arrest decision tree. *CPR,* Cardiopulmonary resuscitation; *ET,* endotracheal; *IO,* intraosseous; *IV,* intravenous. (From the Emergency Cardiac Care Committee and Subcommittee of the American Heart Association, *JAMA* 268:2662, 1992.)
See *Primary Pediatric Care,* ed 3, p. 1796.

- Assess ABCs
- Secure airway
- Administer 100% oxygen
- Start IV or IO access
- Assess vital signs

Severe Cardiorespiratory Compromise?
- Poor perfusion
- Hypotension
- Respiratory difficulty

No

Yes

- Observe
- Support ABCs
- Consider transfer or transport to ALS facility

Perform chest compression if despite oxygenation and ventilation:
- Heart rate <80/min in an infant
- Heart rate <60/min in a child
(Special conditions may apply in the presence of severe hypothermia)

- *Epinephrine*
  - IV/IO: 0.01 mg/kg (1:10 000)
  - ET: 0.1 mg/kg (1:1000)
    (doses up to 0.2 mg/kg [1:1000] may be effective)
  - Repeat every 3-5 min at the same dose

- *Atropine* 0.02 mg/kg
  Minimum dose: 0.1 mg
  Maximum single dose:
    0.5 mg for child
    1.0 mg for adolescent
  May be repeated in 5 min once

If asystole develops, see decision tree illustration on previous page

Bradycardia decision tree. *ABC*, airway, breathing, and circulation; *ALS*, advanced life support; *ET*; endotracheal; *IO*, intraosseous; *IV*, intravenous. (From the Emergency Cardiac Care Committee and Subcommittee of the American Heart Association, *JAMA* 268:2662, 1992.)
See *Primary Pediatric Care*, ed 3, p. 1796.

Cephalosporins

First generation	Second generation	Third generation
Cefadroxil*	Cefaclor*	Cefepime
Cefazolin	Cefamandole	Cefixime*
Cephalexin*	Cefmetazole	Cefmenoxime
Cephalothin	Cefonicid	Cefoperazone
Cephapirin	Cefotetan	Cefotoxime
Cephradine†	Cefotiam	Cefpodoxime proxetil*
	Cefoxitin	Cefpiramide
	Cefprozil*	Cefsulodin
	Cefuroxime	Ceftazidime
	Cefuroxime axetil*	Ceftizoxime
		Ceftriaxone
		Moxalactam

*Oral.
†Oral and parenteral.

See *Primary Pediatric Care,* ed 3, p. 381.

Fluid therapy for dehydration

Degree of dehydration*	Signs†	Rehydration phase‡ (first 4 hours; repeat until no signs of dehydration remain)	Maintenance phase (until illness resolves)
Mild (6%)	Slightly dry mucous membranes, increased thirst	ORS 60 ml/kg	Breast-feeding, undiluted lactose-free formula, ½-strength cow milk or lactose-containing formula
Moderate (8%)	Sunken eyes, sunken fontanelle, loss of skin turgor, dry mucous membranes, decreased urine output	ORS 80 ml/kg	Same as above
Severe (>10%)	Signs of moderate dehydration plus one or more of the following: rapid thready pulse, hypotension, cyanosis, rapid breathing, delayed capillary refill, markedly reduced or absent urine output, lethargy, coma	IV or IO isotonic fluids (0.9% saline or lactated Ringer), 20 ml/kg; repeat until pulse and state of consciousness return to normal, then 50-100 ml/kg of ORS based on remaining degree of dehydration§	Same as above

*Percent of total body weight lost.

†If no signs of dehydration are present, the rehydration phase may be omitted. Proceed with maintenance therapy and replacement of ongoing losses.

‡In addition to the rehydration amounts shown, replace ongoing stool losses and vomitus with ORS, 10 ml/kg for each diarrheal stool and 5 ml/kg for each episode of vomitus.

§While parenteral access is being sought, nasogastric infusion of ORS may be begun at 30 ml/kg/hr, provided airway protective reflexes remain intact.

See *Primary Pediatric Care*, ed 3, p. 1668.

Management of acute diarrhea

I. Less than 5% dehydration without significant vomiting
   A. Nursing infant may continue breastfeeding—supplement with clear fluids as necessary; discontinue solids.
   B. Formula-fed infant
      1. Discontinue formula and solids.
      2. Begin clear liquids (e.g., carbonated beverages, Kool-Aid, Jell-O water, Gatorade, Pedialyte, Ricelyte, Resol). If intake is good without vomiting, offer fluids every 3 to 4 hours; otherwise, offer small quantities more frequently.
      3. As diarrhea resolves, reinstitute formula half strength at first.
      4. If child tolerates half-strength formula for 12 to 24 hours, then go to full strength.
      5. Solids may be introduced as diarrhea resolves (rice, cereal, bananas, crackers, and mashed potatoes without butter).
      6. If reinstitution of formula is not tolerated, continue clear liquids and then try half-strength lactose-free formula (soy formula).
      7. After improvement in diarrhea, increase solids as tolerated.
      8. Reintroduce lactose in patients on lactose-free diet several days to weeks after resolution, depending on severity of original diarrhea; if not tolerated, continue lactose-free diet for several months.
   C. Avoid diphenoxylate (Lomotil), loperamide (Imodium), paregoric, and anticholinergics.
II. Greater than 5% dehydration: either oral or intravenous rehydration
   A. Oral rehydration therapy
      1. Offer rehydration solution *hourly ad libitum:* 50 to 75 mEq/L sodium, 20 to 25 mEq/L potassium, 30 mEq/L bicarbonate or citrate, remainder of anion as chloride, and 20 g/L glucose.
      2. As the diarrhea slows (usually within 24 to 48 hours), begin one-half strength formula (can be lactose free) and advance to regular diet within 24 hours. For ongoing diarrheal losses, supplement with oral hydration solution.
      3. Infants with signs of shock should be given intravenous Ringer lactate (20 ml/kg body weight per hour) until the blood pressure is normal, followed by oral rehydration solution.
      4. Initial vomiting is not a contraindication to the use of oral rehydration; however, persistent vomiting to the extent of interference with rehydration should lead to the use of intravenous fluids.

See *Primary Pediatric Care,* ed 3, p. 905.

Continued

Management of acute diarrhea—cont'd

B. Intravenous fluids
   1. Replacement of deficit is based on estimated percentage of dehydration or known weight loss and serum sodium.
   2. There may be ongoing loss through stool and vomitus.
   3. Maintenance should be appropriate for size.
C. Give half of fluids in first 8 hours, then remainder over next 16 hours (except with hypernatremia, when fluids should be given uniformly with gradual correction over 48 hours; hypotonic fluid should not be used for hypernatremia).
D. If severe dehydration or shock is present, give isotonic fluid or a colloid (10 to 20 ml/kg body weight, over 1 to 2 hours).
E. Delay giving intravenous potassium until urine output is established.
F. As diarrhea resolves, begin treatment as in those patients with less than 5% dehydration, except avoid lactose.

Solutions commonly used in children who have diarrhea

Solution	Glucose/CHO (g/L)	Sodium (mEq/L)	Base (mEq/L; citrate or HCO_3)	Potassium (mEq/L)	Osmolality (mmol/L)
Physiologically appropriate solutions					
Pedialyte	25	45	30	20	270
Ricelyte	30*	50	30	25	200
Rehydralyte	25	75	30	20	310
WHO/UNICEF ORS	20	90	30	20	310
Physiologically inappropriate solutions					
Cola	700	2	13	0.1	750
Apple juice	690	3	0	32	730
Gatorade	255	20	3	3	330

*Rice syrup solids.

See *Primary Pediatric Care*, ed 3, p. 1669.

Therapy of disseminated intravascular coagulation

Acute DIC

Remove trigger (most important)
Coagulation support

Use fresh frozen plasma to maintain PT under 17 seconds (10 ml/kg will raise coagulation factors by 10% to 20%)

Use cryoprecipitate to maintain fibrinogen over 100 mg/dl (1 bag/5 kg will raise fibrinogen by 100 mg/dl)

Use platelet concentrates to maintain platelet count over 50,000 mm^3 (10 ml/kg will raise platelet count by 75,000 to 100,000 mm^3)

Consider use of low-dose heparin therapy
Consider replacement of AT-III and protein C

Chronic DIC

Treat underlying disease
Administer low-dose heparin to inhibit clotting activation
Consider replacement of antithrombin-III and protein C
Consider antifibrinolytic therapy when fibrinogenolysis predominates-
From Manco-Johnson MJ: *Int J Pediatr Hematol Oncol* 1:1, 1994.

See *Primary Pediatric Care,* ed 3, p. 1679.

Treatment of nonretentive encopresis

Don't give medications
Stop all reminders, lectures, or punishments
Give incentives for BMs into the toilet
For soiling, insist on immediate cleanup
Refer treatment failures

See *Primary Pediatric Care,* ed 3, p. 725.

Treatment of retentive encopresis

Hyperphosphate enemas (two or three) to remove impaction
Mineral oil or lactulose for 3 months to keep the stools soft
Laxatives if stool softeners are ineffective
Sitting on the toilet for 10 minutes three times per day
Nonconstipating, high-fiber diet

See *Primary Pediatric Care,* ed 3, p. 723.

Antibiotic regimens for infective endocarditis prophylaxis

Upper respiratory tract surgical procedures (including oral surgery and dental procedures causing gingival bleeding)

1. Standard regimens
   a. Amoxicillin 50 mg/kg (up to 3 g) po 1 hr before the procedure and ½ the initial dose 6 hr later.
   b. For children unable to take oral medications, parenteral ampicillin 50 mg/kg (up to 2 g) 30 min before the procedure and ½ the initial dose 6 hr later.
2. Regimen for those who have intracardiac prosthetic valves or systemic-pulmonary shunts
   Parenteral ampicillin 50 mg/kg (up to 2 g) plus parenteral gentamicin 2.0 mg/kg (up to 80 mg), given 30 min before the procedure. Oral amoxicillin 25 mg/kg (up to 1.5 g) is given 6 hr after the initial antibiotics, or the parenteral regimen can be repeated 8 hr after the first dose. Many authorities recommend one of the above standard regimens for this high-risk group.
3. Regimen for penicillin-allergic patients
   a. Oral: Erythromycin ethylsuccinate or stearate 20 mg/kg (up to 800 mg of erythromycin ethylsuccinate or ≤1 g of erythromycin stearate) 2 hr before the procedure, followed by ½ the initial dose 6 hr later. Alternative regimen: Clindamycin 10 mg/kg (up to 300 mg) po 1 hr before the procedure, followed by ½ the initial dose 6 hr later.
   b. Parenteral: Clindamycin 10 mg/kg IV (up to 300 mg) 30 min before the procedure, followed by ½ the initial dose 6 hr later.
   c. Parenteral for patients who have intracardiac prosthetic material or systemic-pulmonary shunts: Vancomycin 20 mg/kg IV (up to 1g) given over 1 hr, starting 1 hr before the procedure.

For GI/GU surgical procedures

1. Standard regimen: Parenteral ampicillin and gentamicin 30 to 60 min before the procedure and again 8 hr later. Alternatively, oral amoxicillin may be given 6 hr after the initial antibiotics. Dosages are the same as for upper respiratory tract surgery.
2. Oral regimen for minor procedures in a low-risk patient: Amoxicillin 50 mg/kg (up to 3 g) 1 hr before the procedure and ½ the initial dose 6 hr later.
3. Regimen for penicillin-allergic patients: IV vancomycin and gentamicin 1 hr before the procedure, with a repeat dose 8 hr later. Dosages are the same as given for upper respiratory tract surgical procedures.

See *Primary Pediatric Care*, ed 3, p. 103.

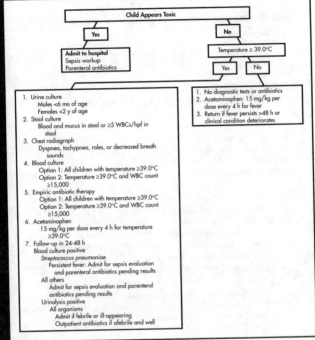

Algorithm for the management of a previously healthy child 91 days to 36 months of age with fever without source. (From Baroff LJ et al: *Pediatrics* 92:1, 1993.)
See *Primary Pediatric Care*, ed 3, p. 963.

Fever without source, infant

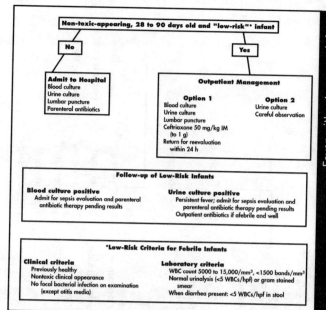

Algorithm for the management of a previously healthy infant 0 to 90 days of age with fever without source ≥ 38.0° C. (From Baroff LJ et al: *Pediatrics* 92:1, 1993.)

See *Primary Pediatric Care*, ed 3, p. 963.

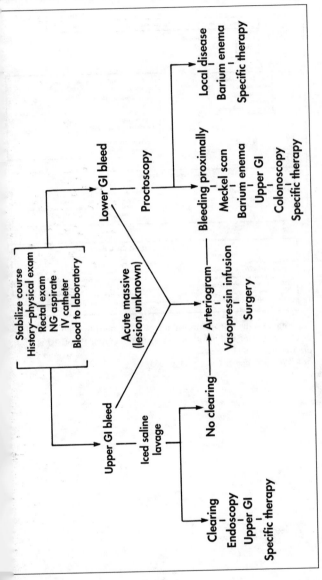

Management of gastrointestinal hemorrhage.
See *Primary Pediatric Care*, ed 3, p. 982.

Heart failure

Initial therapy in heart failure

Therapy	Route	Dosage	Onset of action
Oxygen	Nasal, endotracheal tube	40%-100%	Immediate
Furosemide	IV, PO	1-2 mg/kg	15-30 min
Digoxin	IV, PO	5-10 µg/kg	5-30 min
Dopamine	IV	5-20 µg/kg/min	Immediate
Dobutamine	IV	5-20 µg/kg/min	Immediate

See *Primary Pediatric Care,* ed 3, p. 1713.

High blood pressure

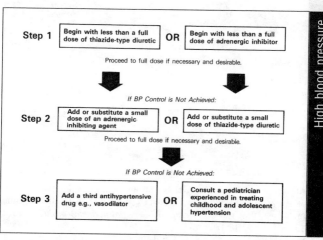

Stepped-care approach to antihypertensive drug therapy. (From Task Force on Blood Pressure Control in Children: *Pediatrics* 79:1, 1987; courtesy Dr. Michael J. Horan.)
See *Primary Pediatric Care,* ed 3, p. 1013.

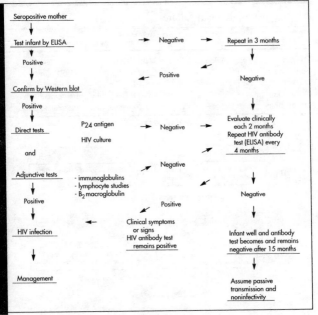

Algorithm for determining whether an infant has HIV infection or only passively acquired antibodies. (From Dossett JH: Perinatal HIV infection. In Nelson NM: *Current therapy in neonatal-perinatal medicine,* ed 2, Toronto, 1989, BC Decker.)

See *Primary Pediatric Care,* ed 3, p. 1175.

Treatment of hyperkalemia in pediatric patients

Agent	Dose	Effect	Remarks
Calcium gluconate (10%)	0.5 ml/kg IV over 2-4 min	Rapid but transient	Monitor ECG for bradycardia during injection; may be repeated but *not likely* to be effective
Sodium bicarbonate (7.5%)	2.5 mEq/kg (approximately 3 ml/kg) IV by slow push	Rapid but transient	Repetition *not* recommended
Glucose (50%)	1 ml/kg IV by slow push	Within 1-2 hr	Attempt to increase blood glucose to 250 mg/dl; may be maintained by infusion of 30% glucose at rate equal to insensible fluid loss
Insulin (regular)	0.1 U/kg IV	Rapid	Give *only* with hypertonic glucose infusion (30%)
Sodium polystyrene sulfonate (Kayexalate)	1 g/kg PO or PR	Hours to days	Side effects: gastric irritation (nausea and vomiting), diarrhea, *or* fecal impaction; PO more effective than PR; enemas should be retained 4-10 hr for effectiveness—removed by cleansing enema; may cause *hypokalemia*; use cautiously in patients who tolerate sodium loads poorly; also chelates Ca^{++} and Mg^{++}

See *Primary Pediatric Care,* ed 3, p. 1760.

Dose of L-thyroxine in treating hypothyroidism

Age	T_4 dose per day (μg)	T_4 dose/kg/day (μg)
<6 mo	25-50	8-10
6-12 mo	50-75	6-8
1-5 yr	75-100	5-6
6-12 yr	100-125	4-5
>12 yr	100-200	2-3

See *Primary Pediatric Care,* ed 3, p. 1361.

Initial empirical therapy for selected infections*

Clinical diagnosis	Most likely offending organisms	Antimicrobial agents
Meningitis	**Neonate:** group B streptococci, E. coli, L. monocytogenes	Ampicillin and cefotaxime (or ceftriaxone)
	Child: S. pneumoniae, N. meningitidis, H. influenzae type b	Ceftriaxone or cefotaxime (plus vancomycin if S. pneumoniae is suspected)
Brain abscess	Streptococcal species, anaerobes, S. aureus	Penicillin and metronidazole (plus nafcillin if S. aureus is suspected)
Orbital cellulitis	Streptococcal species, S. aureus, H. influenzae type b	Ceftriaxone or cefotaxime plus clindamycin
Epiglottitis	H. influenzae type b	Ceftriaxone or cefotaxime
Pneumonia (lobar or segmental)	**Neonate:** group B streptococci, S. aureus, gram negative organisms	Ampicillin plus an aminoglycoside
	Child: S. pneumoniae, H. influenzae type b, S. aureus, S. pyogenes, M. pneumoniae	Penicillin or nafcillin, or erythromycin
Infective endocarditis	Streptococcus viridans, S. aureus	Nafcillin plus an aminoglycoside
Acute diarrhea (fecal WBC present)	Salmonella, Shigella species	If patient is systemically ill, very young, or immunocompromised, cefotaxime or ceftriaxone
Abdominal sepsis	Anaerobes, aerobic enterics, enterococci	Clindamycin, aminoglycoside, and ampicillin
Urinary tract infection	**Acute:** E. coli, Klebsiella species	Gentamicin or trimethoprim/sulfamethoxazole (TMP-SMX)
	Chronic: E. coli, Proteus species, Pseudomonas species	Await culture and sensitivity results

See *Primary Pediatric Care*, ed 3, p. 391.

Osteomyelitis	**Neonate:** group B streptococci, *S. aureus, S. pyogenes, S. pneumoniae*	Nafcillin plus an aminoglycoside
	Child: *S. aureus, S. pyogenes*	Nafcillin
Pyogenic arthritis	**Neonate:** group B streptococci, *S. aureus, S. pyogenes, N. gonorrhoea*	Nafcillin and an aminoglycoside
	Child: *H. influenzae* type b (<5 yr), *S. aureus, S. pyogenes, N. gonorrhoea*	Ceftriaxone or cefotaxime (test MIC for *S. aureus*) plus nafcillin
Suspected sepsis	**Neonate:** group B streptococci, *L. monocytogenes*, gram negative enteric organisms	Ampicillin plus an aminoglycoside
	Infant (1-6 wk): as for neonate plus as for child	Ampicillin plus ceftriaxone
	Child: *S. pneumoniae, H. influenzae* type b, *N. meningitidis*	Ceftriaxone
Compromised host		
Fever only		Cefotaxime or aminopenicillin
Pneumonia	*S. aureus, E. coli, Pseudomonas* species	As under pneumonia above plus TMP-SMX; if patient's condition deteriorates, bronchoalveolar lavage (BAL) or lung biopsy is needed to direct therapy
	As under pneumonia above, and *P. carinii, Candida albicans*, other fungi	
Shock (sepsis without source)	**Neonate:** group B streptococci, enterics	Ampicillin plus an aminoglycoside
	Child: *N. meningitidis, S. pneumoniae*	Ceftriaxone or cefotaxime

*For most clinical diagnoses, an acceptable alternative choice of antibiotics could be proposed.

Chelation therapy of lead poisoning

Status	Therapy	Comments
Encephalopathy	BAL* 75 mg/m² IM every 4 hr for 5 days CaEDTA† 1500 mg/m²/day IV over 6 hr for 5 days	Give BAL 4 hr before CaEDTA infusion. Treat 5 additional days (after 2-day break) if PbB remains high. Additional cycles may be necessary depending on PbB rebound.
PbB of 70 µg/dl or higher or nonencephalopathic symptomatology	BAL 50 mg/m² IM every 4 hr for 3-5 days CaEDTA 1000 mg/m²/day IV over 6 yr for 5 days	Give BAL 4 hr before CaEDTA infusion. BAL may be stopped after 3 days if the PbB falls below 50 µg/dl. Additional cycles may be necessary depending on PbB rebound.
PbB of 50 µg/dl or higher under 70 µg/dl PbB of 25 µg/dl or higher under 50 µg/dl	CaEDTA 1000 mg/m²/day IV over 6 hr for 5 days	Additional cycles may be necessary depending on PbB rebound.

Adapted from Piomelli S et al: *J Pediatr* 105:527, 1984.
*Medicinal iron should not be given concurrently with BAL therapy.
†Adequate diuresis is essential (IV or oral fluid) to minimize renal toxicity.

See *Primary Pediatric Care*, ed 3, p. 1749.

Approach to acute management of leukemia

A. Initial evaluation

History—Fatigue, malaise, anorexia, irritability, fever, bone pain, mouth sores

Physical examination—Pallor, petechiae, purpura, fever, lymphadenopathy, hepatosplenomegaly, respiratory distress, neurological abnormalities

Laboratory—Complete blood count with differential and platelet count, abnormal results of one or more cell lines

B. Suspicion of leukemia as a possible diagnosis and potential emergency interventions

Findings	Management
1. Temperature over 100.4° F (38° C), neutrophil count <500; symptoms of infection	Blood culture, antibiotics
2. Bleeding symptoms	Start intravenous unit for access and delivery of a fluid bolus, transfuse platelets, red cells, or plasma
3. Respiratory distress	Chest roentgenogram, oxygen
4. WBC >100,000	Blood urea nitrogen and creatinine, urate, serum potassium, serum calcium, serum phosphate, chest roentgenogram, start intravenous unit for access and delivery of a fluid bolus

C. Refer patient to a pediatric oncology center

Consult with a pediatric oncologist

Arrange for transfer of patient to the pediatric oncology center

Prepare patient and family for what to expect when they get there

See *Primary Pediatric Care*, ed 3, p. 1403.

Treatment regimens for Lyme disease

Manifestation	Regimen*
Early infection*	
Adults	Tetracycline, 250 mg orally 4× daily, 10-30 days†
	Doxycycline, 100 mg orally 2× daily, 10-30 days†‡
	Amoxicillin, 500 mg orally 4× daily, 10-30 days†‡
Children (≤8 yr)	Amoxicillin or penicillin V, 250 mg orally 3× daily or 25-50 mg/kg body weight/day in 3 divided doses, 10-30 days
	In case of penicillin allergy:
	Erythromycin, 250 mg orally 3× daily or 30 mg/kg/day in divided doses, 10-30 days‡
Neurological abnormalities (early or late)*	
General	Ceftriaxone, 75-100 mg/kg/day intravenously 1× daily, 14 days§
	Penicillin G, 300,000 U/kg/day intravenously, 6 divided doses daily, 14 days§
	In case of ceftriaxone or penicillin allergy:
	Doxycycline, 100 mg orally 2× daily, 30 days‡
	Chloramphenicol, 250 mg intravenously 4× daily, 14 days‡
Facial palsy alone	Oral antibiotic regimens may be adequate
Cardiac abnormalities	
First-degree atrioventricular block (PR interval <0.3 sec)	Oral antibiotic regimens, as for early infection
High-degree atrioventricular block	Ceftriaxone, 75-100 mg/kg/day intravenously 1× daily, 14 days‡
	Penicillin, 300,000 U/kg/day intravenously, 6 divided doses daily, 14 days‡
Arthritis (intermittent or chronic)†	Doxycycline, 100 mg orally 2× daily, 30 days
	Amoxicillin and probenecid, 500 mg each orally 4× daily, 30 days
	Ceftriaxone, 75-100 mg/kg/day intravenously 1× daily, 14 days
	Penicillin, 300,000 U/kg/day intravenously, 6 divided doses daily, 14 days
Acrodermatitis	Oral antibiotic regimens for 1 mo usually are adequate

Adapted from Steere AC: *N Engl J Med* 321:586, 1989.

*Treatment failures have occurred with all these regimens, and retreatment may be necessary.
†The duration of therapy is based on the clinical response.
‡The antibiotic has not yet been tested systematically for this indication in Lyme disease.
§The appropriate duration of therapy is not yet clear for patients with late neurological abnormalities, and it may be longer than 2 weeks.

See *Primary Pediatric Care*, ed 3, p. 1417.

Antibiotic treatment of acute otitis media

Drug	Common trade name(s)	Dose/day (mg/kg)	Dose frequency/day
Amoxicillin	Amoxil, Polymox	20–40	×3
Amoxicillin-potassium clavulanate	Augmentin	40/10	×3
Cefaclor	Ceclor	40	×2
Cefixime	Suprax	8	×1
Cefprozil	Cefzil	15	×2
Cefuroxime axetil	Ceftin	15	×2
Erythromycin-sulfisoxazole	Pediazole	50/150	×2
Loracarbef	Lorabid	30	×4
Trimethoprim-sulfamethoxazole	Bactrim, Septra	8/40	×2

See *Primary Pediatric Care*, ed 3, p. 1473.

Postexposure antirabies treatment guide*

Species of animal	Animal's condition at time of attack	Treatment of exposed person
Wild skunk, fox, coyote, raccoon, or bat	Regard as rabid	HDCV† and RIG
Domestic dog or cat	Healthy	None‡
	Unknown (escaped)	Call public health official
	Rabid or suspected of being rabid	HDCV and RIG‡
Other	Consider individually	

Modified from the Report of the Committee on Infectious Diseases *Red book*, ed 19, Evanston, Ill, 1982, American Academy of Pediatrics.

HDCV, Human diploid cell (rabies) vaccine; *RIG*, (Human) rabies immune globulin.

*These recommendations are only guidelines; they should be applied in conjunction with information about the species of animal involved, the circumstances of the bite or nonbite exposure, the animal's vaccination status, and whether rabies is present in the region.

†The vaccine is discontinued if the animal is killed at the time of the attack and subsequent fluorescent antibody tests are negative for rabies.

‡HDCV and RIG are begun at the first sign of rabies in a biting dog or cat during the 10-day holding period.

See *Primary Pediatric Care*, ed 3, p. 191.

Rabies vaccination guidelines

Animal	Management
Wild carnivores	Begin HRIG and HDCV. Submit animal's head for testing.
Healthy domestic dogs and cats	Quarantine animal; treat only if animal develops symptoms.
Stray or sick dogs and cats	Submit animal's head for testing. Delay treatment until test results are known unless clinical likelihood of rabies is high. If animal is unavailable, complete full series of HRIG and HDCV.
Rodents, rabbits	Unlikely to be rabid (except woodchucks). Treat only if animal acted strangely and cannot be tested.

From Schmidt MJ, Olson JG, Krebs JW: *Contemp Pediatr* 10:36, 1993.

See *Primary Pediatric Care*, ed 3, p. 1183.

Management of staphylococcal toxic shock syndrome

1. Consider other possible diagnoses
2. Remove potentially infected foreign bodies (e.g., tampons)
3. Obtain cultures of blood, throat, vagina, nares, rectum, and other appropriate sites
4. Drain and irrigate infected sites
5. Give an intravenous antistaphylococcal beta-lactamase-resistant antimicrobial agent at maximum dosage for weight and age
6. Consider methylprednisolone for severe cases
7. Treat aggressively and monitor for the following:
   Hypovolemia and inadequate tissue perfusion
   Adult respiratory distress syndrome
   Myocardial dysfunction
   Acute renal failure
   Cerebral edema
   Hypocalcemia/hypophosphatemia
   Metabolic acidosis
   Disseminated intravascular coagulation
   Fluid and electrolyte abnormalities

Staphylococcal toxic shock syndrome

See *Primary Pediatric Care,* ed 3, p. 1614.

Treatment of status epilepticus

A. Assess cardiovascular function by making sure the airway is clear and the patient is breathing. Provide oxygen or respiratory support as necessary.

B. Establish an intravenous line and obtain blood samples for electrolytes, blood urea nitrogen, calcium, a complete blood count, and anticonvulsant medication levels. A blood Dextrostix test should be performed immediately, and if the glucose is under 60 mg%, then 1 to 2 ml/kg of D25W should be administered.

C. One member of the emergency team should obtain a history while another does a brief physical examination.

D. Administer anticonvulsant drugs in the following order until seizure activity is controlled:

1. Initial therapy

   a. Lorazepam should be the initial anticonvulsant administered intravenously at a dose of 0.1 mg/kg (maximum 4 mg) over 2 minutes; a dose of 0.05 to 0.1 mg/kg may be repeated every 5 minutes if necessary up to a maximum of 0.5 mg/kg, but not over 10 mg in toto.

   b. If lorazepam is not available, diazepam should be administered intravenously at a dose of 0.1 to 0.2 mg/kg (maximum 10 mg) by "pushing" half the dose over 1 minute and the remainder at 1 mg/minute. A dose of 0.1 mg/kg may be repeated in 5 minutes if necessary. Because of diazepam's short duration of anticonvulsant effect, another anticonvulsant such as phenytoin must be administered immediately.

   c. If the patient is known to be receiving phenytoin on a chronic basis, it should be administered as the initial anticonvulsant (see D.2.).

2. If status epilepticus continues, administer phenytoin 15 to 20 mg/kg intravenously up to a total dose of 1000 mg. A quarter of the dose may be administered during the first 2 minutes and then at a rate of 1 to 2 mg/kg/minute (maximum rate of 50 mg/minute). If the patient is known to be receiving phenytoin chronically, 5 to 8 mg/kg of phenytoin may be administered as the initial anticonvulsant. Monitor the heart rate, and slow the rate of phenytoin infusion if bradycardia occurs. If seizure activity continues despite a full loading dose of phenytoin, correct for presumed acidosis with a modest dose of sodium bicarbonate.

3. If status epilepticus continues, administer phenobarbital 15 to 20 mg/kg intravenously up to a total dose of 800 mg. Administer phenobarbital over 15 minutes, monitoring respirations and blood pressure, especially if the patient has been given a benzodiazepine.

4. If status epilepticus persists, administer paraldehyde 0.3 ml/kg mixed with mineral oil (maximum of 5 ml) per rectum.

E. If seizure activity still persists, consult a neurologist to determine the need for other anticonvulsants, general anesthesia, or induction of pentobarbital coma.

See *Primary Pediatric Care*, ed 3, p. 1774.

Medication Comparison Tables

Analgesic medications

Agonist	Equipotent IV dose (mg/kg)	Duration (hr)	Bioavailability (%)	Comments
Morphine	0.1	3-4	20-40	Seizures in newborns and in all patients at high doses Histamine release, vasodilation—avoid in asthmatics and in circulatory compromise MS Contin 8-12 hr duration
Meperidine	1	3-4	40-60	Catastrophic interactions with MAO inhibitors Tachycardia; negative inotrope Metabolite produces seizures; not recommended for chronic use
Methadone	0.1	6-24	70-100	Can be given IV even though the package insert says SQ or IM
Fentanyl	0.001	0.5-1		Bradycardia; minimal hemodynamic alterations Chest wall rigidity (>5 µg/kg rapid IV bolus). R_X naloxone or a succinylcholine, pancuronium
Codeine	1.2	3-4	40-70	PO only Prescribe with acetaminophen
Oxycodone (Tylox, Percocet)	0.05-0.15	3-4	40-60	PO primarily Prescribed with acetaminophen
Hydromorphone (Dilaudid)	0.015-0.02	3-4	40-60	<CNS depression than morphine <Itching and nausea than morphine Can be used in PCA

See *Primary Pediatric Care*, ed 3, p. 1529.

Common antiarrhythmic agents

Drugs	Initial therapy	Maintenance therapy	Toxic effects
Digoxin	Digitalization 20-40 µg/kg divided in four equal doses	PO, 1/4 digitalizing dose/day	Heart block, ectopy
Quinidine	PO, 2 mg/kg every test dose	PO, 4-10 mg/kg every 6 hr	Rash, fever, gastrointestinal (GI) symptoms, purpura, hemolytic anemia, hypotension
Procainamide	IV, 2 mg/kg of 1:10 dilution over 5 minutes	PO, 5-15 mg/kg every 6 hr	Lupuslike syndrome, hypotension, urticaria, GI symptoms
Lidocaine	IV, 1 mg/kg of 1:1000 dilution over 3-5 minutes; up to 5 mg/kg	IV, 0.03 mg/kg/minute of dilute solution of 5 mg/ml; decrease rate as arrhythmia continues to be controlled	Convulsions, drowsiness, euphoria, muscle twitching
Phenytoin	IV, 10-15 mg/kg over 5 minutes	PO, 2 mg/kg tid	Hypotension, ataxia
Propranolol	IV, 0.01-0.15 mg/kg over 3-5 minutes	PO, 0.05-1 mg/kg/day divided, every 6 hr	Bradycardia, hypotension, cardiac failure, asthma
Isoproterenol	IV, 0.1-1.0 µg/kg/minute	Infusion adjusted to maintain stable rhythm and rate	Ventricular ectopic beats, tachycardia
Atropine	IV, 0.01-0.03 mg/kg (0.15 mg minimum; 0.5 mg maximum flushing)		Mydriasis, dry mouth
Adenosine	IV, 0.05-0.25 mg/kg/dose IV push	None	Blocks AV node conduction to convert SVT

See *Primary Pediatric Care*, ed 3, p. 886.

Medications used to treat children who have asthma

Drug	Formulation/administration	Dose/duration
Bronchodilators		
Sympathomimetics		
Epinephrine		
Epinephrine	1:1000 solution SQ	0.01 ml/kg up to 0.33 ml
Sus-Phrine*	1:200 suspension, SQ	0.005 ml/kg up to 0.25 ml
Albuterol		
Proventil*	Metered aerosol	90 µg/puff
Ventolin*	Tablet: 2, 4 mg	0.1 mg/kg tid
	Syrup: 2 mg/5 ml	0.1 mg/kg tid
	Aerosol solution: 1%	0.5 ml/2.5 ml saline
Metaproterenol		
Alupent*	Aerosol solution: 5%	0.25 ml/2.5 ml saline
Metaprel*	Metered aerosol	650 µg/puff
	Syrup: 10 mg/5 ml	0.5 mg/kg tid
	Tablet: 10, 20 mg	0.5 mg/kg tid
Terbutaline		
Brethine*	Solution SQ	0.25 ml/dose
Bricanyl*	Tablet: 2.5, 5 mg	0.075 mg/kg tid
Theophyllines†		
Theo-Dur Sprinkle*	Capsule: 50, 75, 125 mg	q8-12h (long duration)
Theo-Dur*	Tablet: 100, 200, 300 mg	q8-12h (long duration)
Slo-Phyllin*	Gyrocap: 60, 125, 200 mg	q8-12h (long duration)
Slo-Bid*	Gyrocap: 100, 200, 300 mg	q8-12h (long duration)
Antiinflammatory drugs		
Cromolyn	Aerosol solution: 2 µg/2 ml	20 g qid
	Metered aerosol	2 puffs qid
Nedocromil	Metered aerosol	2 puffs qid
Inhaled corticosteroids		
Beclomethasone (Vanceril,* Beclovent*)	Metered aerosol	44 mg/puff
Triamcinolone (Azmacort*)	Metered aerosol	100 mg/puff
Flunisolide (AeroBid*)	Metered aerosol	250 mg/puff

*Trade name.
†The normal dosage (12-16 mg/kg/24 hr) must be individualized.

See *Primary Pediatric Care*, ed 3, p. 1192.

Dosage guidelines for commonly used antiemetics

Pharmacological group (generic)	Brand name	Dosage (mg/kg)	Comments
Phenothiazines			
Chlorpromazine	Thorazine	IV, PO: 0.5-1 q6-8 hr	Adverse effects include drowsiness, hypotension, arrhythmias, extrapyramidal symptoms; potentiates effects of opioids, sedatives
Prochlorperazine	Compazine	PO, PR: 0.1 q6-8 hr (max 10 mg)	
Butyrophenones			
Droperidol	Inapsine	IV: 0.01-0.03 q6-8 hr	Adverse effects include drowsiness, hypotension, arrhythmias, extrapyramidal symptoms; lowers seizure threshold; potentiates effects of opioids, sedatives
Haloperidol	Haldol	IV: 0.01 q8-12 hr	
Antihistamines			
Promethazine	Phenergan	IV: 0.25-0.5 q6 hr	Adverse effects include drowsiness, hypotension, arrhythmias; contraindicated in patients taking MAO inhibitors
Diphenhydramine	Benadryl	0.5-1.0 q4-6 hr (max 50 mg)	
Benzamides			
Metoclopramide	Reglan	IV, PO: 0.05-0.1 q6 hr	Adverse effects include extrapyramidal symptoms
Anticholinergics			
Scopolamine	Hyoscine, transdermal scopolamine	IV, PO: 0.005 q4-6 hr apply behind ear 4 hr before needed; lasts 72 hr	Adverse effects include dry mouth, blurred vision, fever, tachycardia, constipation, urinary retention, drowsiness, amnesia
Antiserotonin			
Ondansetron	Zofran	IV, PO: 0.15 q8hr, (max dose 4 mg)	Adverse effects include bronchospasm, tachycardia, headaches, lightheadedness

See *Primary Pediatric Care*, ed 3, p. 1524.

Common antiepileptic medications

Drug	Indications	Half-life (hours)	Usual dose (mg/kg/day)	Therapeutic levels (μg/ml)	Adverse effects
Carbamazepine	Partial, secondary generalized	3-23 (18-55 initially)	5-25 5-10 (monotherapy)	4-12	Allergic rashes, nausea, diplopia, blurry vision, dizziness, hypersensitivity hepatitis, aplastic anemia
Phenytoin	Partial, secondary generalized, primary generalized	7-42 (nonlinear kinetics)	5-7	10-20 (occasionally lower)	Rashes, hirsutism, gingival hyperplasia, coarse features, psychomotor slowing, neuropathy, folate deficiency, myelosuppression, drug-induced lupus
Valproic acid	Primary generalized, absence, myoclonic, akinetic, febrile, infantile spasms, some partial	6-16	10-30 20-50 (infants and in polytherapy)	50-100 (150 if tolerated)	Nausea, tremor, weight gain, hair loss, thrombocytopenia, hepatic failure, pancreatitis
Phenobarbital	Neonatal, febrile, partial, secondary generalized, primary generalized, akinetic	36-120	3-5 (<25 kg) 2-3 (25-50 kg) 1-2 (>50 kg)	10-40	Sedation, inattention, hyperactivity, irritability, cognitive impairment, rare hypersensitivity reactions
Ethosuximide	Absence, myoclonic, akinetic	15-68	15-40	40-100	Nausea, abdominal discomfort, hiccups, drowsiness, behavioral problems, dystonias, myelosuppression, drug-induced lupus

					Adverse effects
Primidone	Partial, secondary generalized, primary generalized	3-20	5-10 (1-2 initially)	5-12	Sedation, irritability, psychomotor slowing, rare hematological and hypersensitivity reactions
Clonazepam	Absence, primary generalized, infantile spasms	20-36	0.01-0.2	0.01-0.07	Sedation, hyperactivity, inattention, aggressiveness, tolerance, ataxia, withdrawal seizures
Acetazolamide	Absence, myoclonic, akinetic, partial	10-12	10-20	10-14	Diuresis, paresthesias, sedation, CO_2 retention, rashes
Felbamate	Partial (in patients >12 years), Lennox-Gastaut syndrome	20 (in monotherapy)	15-45 (maximum of 3600 mg)	—	Anorexia, weight loss, nausea, insomnia, headache, fatigue, aplastic anemia
Gabapentin	Partial, with or without secondary generalized seizures in patients >12 years	5-7	Total daily dose 900-1800 mg	—	Somnolence, dizziness, ataxia, fatigue
Lamotrigine	Partial, primary generalized, absence, atypical absence, atonic, and myoclonic	7 to 45	5-15 without valproic acid, 1-5 with valproic acid	—	

See *Primary Pediatric Care*, ed 3, p. 1570.

Recommended doses of parenteral and oral antifungal drugs

Drug	Route	Dose (per day)	Adverse reactions*
Amphotericin B	IV	0.25 mg/kg (after test dose†) initially, increase as tolerated to 0.5-1 mg/kg; infuse as single dose over 4-6 hr	Fever, chills, phlebitis, renal dysfunction, hypokalemia, anemia, cardiac arrhythmias, anaphylactoid reaction, hematological abnormalities
	Intrathecal (IT)	0.025 mg, increase to 0.1-0.5 mg twice weekly	Radiculitis, sensory loss, foot drop
Clotrimazole (troches)	PO (topical)	10 mg tablet 5 times/day (dissolved slowly in the mouth)	Nausea, vomiting, increase in serum transaminase
Fluconazole	IV	*Children‡:* 3-6 mg/kg/day	Rash, nausea, abdominal pain, diarrhea, headache, possibly hepatotoxicity
	PO	*Adults:* 200 mg once, followed by 100 mg/day for oropharyngeal, esophageal candidiasis; 400 mg once, followed by 200-400 mg/day for cryptococcal meningitis (200 mg/day for maintenance in patients with acquired immune deficiency syndrome [AIDS])	
Flucytosine	PO	50-150 mg/kg in 4 doses at 6-hr intervals (adjust dosage with renal dysfunction)	Bone marrow suppression; renal dysfunction can lead to drug accumulation; nausea, vomiting, increases in transaminases, blood urea nitrogen (BUN), and creatinine

*See the package insert or the listing in the current edition of the *Physicians' Desk Reference*, Montvale, NJ, Medical Economics.

†Test dose is 0.1 mg/kg, with a maximum dose of 1 mg/kg.

‡The daily dose has not been established for children ≤2 yr.

Drug	Route	Dose	Side Effects
Griseofulvin	PO	Ultramicrosize: 7.3 mg/kg, single dose; maximum dose, 375-750 mg Microsize: 15-20 mg/kg/day divided in 2 doses; maximum dose, 500-1000 mg	Rash, leukopenia, proteinuria, paresthesia, GI symptoms, mental confusion
Itraconazole	PO	*Children:* dose has not been established; a dose of 100 mg/day has been reported for children 3-16 yr *Adults:* 200 mg once or twice daily	Nausea, epigastric pain, headache, edema, hypokalemia, increased serum aminotransferase, hypertension, adrenal insufficiency
Ketoconazole	PO	*Children:* 3.3-6.6 mg/kg, once daily§ *Adults:* 200-400 mg once daily	Rash, anaphylaxis, nausea, vomiting, abdominal pain, fever, gynecomastia, thrombocytopenia, hepatoxicity, and depression of endocrine function (dose dependent, reversible); should not be given concurrently with the antihistamine terfenadine
Miconazole	IV	20-40 mg/kg/day divided into 3 infusions 8 hr apart; maximum 15 mg/kg per infusion; infuse over 30-60 min	Phlebitis, rash, fever, nausea, anemia, hyponatremia, thrombocytopenia, hyperlipemia
	IT	20 mg per dose for 3-7 days	
Nystatin	PO	*Infants:* 200,000 U 4 times/day *Children and adults:* 400,000-600,000 U 4 times/day	Nausea, vomiting, diarrhea

§Efficacy has not been established for children. A small number of children 3 to 13 years of age have been treated safely with this dose.

See *Primary Pediatric Care,* ed l3, p. 392.

Antihypertensive medications*

	Dose	Times/day	Route
Diuretics			
Hydrochlorothiazide (Hydrodiuril, Esidrix)	1-2 mg/kg	2	Oral
Chlorthalidone (Hygroton)	0.5-2 mg/kg	1	Oral
Furosemide (Lasix)	0.5-2 mg/kg	2	Oral, intravenous (IV)
Spironolactone (Aldactone)	1-2 mg/kg	2	Oral
Triamterene (Dyrenium)	1-2 mg/kg	2	Oral
Adrenergic inhibitors			
Beta-adrenergic antagonists			
Metoprolol (Lopressor)	1-4 mg/kg	2	Oral
Atenolol (Tenormin)	1-2 mg/kg	1	Oral
Propranolol (Inderal)	1-3 mg/kg	3	Oral
Central adrenergic inhibitors			
Methyldopa (Aldomet)	5-10 mg/kg	2	Oral
Clonidine (Catapres)	0.05-0.40 mg	2	Oral
Guanabenz (Wytensin)	0.03-0.08 mg	2	Oral
Alpha-adrenergic antagonist			
Prazosin hydrochloride (Minipress)	0.5-7 mg	3	Oral
Vasodilators			
Hydralazine (Apresoline)	1-5 mg/kg	2 or 3	Oral, intramuscular, IV (drip)
Minoxidil (Loniten)	0.1-1.0 mg/kg	2	Oral
Diazoxide (Hyperstat)†	3-5 mg/kg/dose		IV (bolus)
Nitroprusside (Nipride)†	1-8 µg/kg/minute		IV (drip)
Angiotensin-converting enzyme inhibitor			
Captopril			
≤6 mo of age	0.05-0.5 mg/kg	3	Oral
≥6 mo of age	0.5-2 mg/kg	3	Oral

Adapted from Task Force on Blood Pressure Control in Children: *Pediatrics* 79:1, 1987; courtesy Dr. Michael J. Horan.

*Not to exceed usual adult dosage with all drugs.

†Primary use is in hypertensive emergencies.

See *Primary Pediatric Care,* ed 3, p. 1012.

Dosage, peak serum concentrations, and MIC$_{95}$ for selected antimicrobial agents

Antimicrobial agent (route)	Age				Peak serum concentration ($\mu g/ml$)	Susceptibility (MIC$_{95}$) ($\mu g/ml$)‡
	<1 wk* (<2000 g) mg/kg/dose/interval	1 wk-1 mo* (<2000 g) mg/kg/dose/interval	>1 mo mg/kg/dose/interval	Adult dose† g/dose/interval		
Penicillin G (IV)	50,000 U q6h (50,000 U q12h)	50,000 U q6h (50,000 U q8h)	25,000-50,000 U q4-6h	25,000-50,000 U/kg q4-6h	400	≤0.1 L. monocytogenes ≤2
Procaine penicillin (IM)	50,000 U q24h (50,000 U q24h)	50,000 U q24h (50,000 U q24h)	25,000-50,000 U q12-24h	25,000-50,000 U/kg q12-24h	5-6	≤0.1
Benzathine I penicillin (IM)	50,000 U; 1 dose (50,000 U; 1 dose)	50,000 U; 1 dose (50,000 U; 1 dose)	50,000 U; 1 dose	2.4 × 10⁶ U; 1 dose	0.2	≤0.1
Penicillin V (PO)	Not recommended	Not recommended			3-5	≤0.1
Ampicillin (IV, IM)	25-50 q8h (25-50 q12h)	25-50 q6h (25-50 q8h)	6.25-12.5 q6h 25-75 q4-6h	0.25-0.5 q6h 1-2 q4-6h	40 8	Gram negative ≤8 Streptococci ≤0.1 H. influenzae ≤2
Amoxicillin (PO)	Not recommended	Not recommended	10-15 q8h	0.25-0.5 q8h	4.7-7.5	As for ampicillin
Nafcillin (IV)	20 q8h (25 q12h)	37.5 q6h (25 q8h)	25-50 q6h	0.5-1.5 q4-6h	11	≤1
Methicillin§ (IV)	25-50 q8h (25-50 q12h)	25-50 q6h (25-50 q8h)	—	—	—	—
Dicloxacillin (PO)	Not recommended	Not recommended	3-6.25	0.25-0.5 q6h	15-18	≤1

*Doses and intervals shown in parentheses are for infants with a birth weight <2000 g; doses and intervals shown without parentheses are for infants with a birth weight >2000 g.
†Maximum recommended dose (units other than grams are in **boldface**).
‡$\mu g/ml$ of the antimicrobial required to inhibit isolate reported to be susceptible to disk diffusion method.
§Methicillin is preferred for newborns when kernicterus is a concern.

Continued.

Dosage, peak serum concentrations, and MIC$_{95}$ for selected antimicrobial agents—cont'd

| Antimicrobial agent (route) | Age | | | Adult dose† g/dose/interval | Peak serum concentration (μg/ml) | Susceptibility (MIC$_{95}$) (μg/ml)‡ |
	<1 wk* (<2000 g) mg/kg/dose/interval	1 wk-1 mo* (<2000 g) mg/kg/dose/interval	>1 mo mg/kg/dose/interval			
Mezlocillin (IV, IM)	75 q12h (75 q12h)	75 q8h (75 q8h)	50-75 q4-6h	3-4 q4-6h	200-300	≤64
Cefazolin (IV, IM)	20 q12h (20 q12h)	20 q8h (20 q12h)	8.3-25 q6-8h	0.5-1.5 q6-8h	188	≤8
Cephalexin (PO)	Not recommended	Not recommended	6.25-12.5 q6h	0.25-1 q6h	8-40	≤8
Cefoxitin (IV, IM)	Not recommended	Not recommended	20-26.6 q4-q6h	1-2 q4-q6h or 3 q8h	110-125	≤8
Cefotaxime (IV)	50 q8h (50 q12h)	50 q8h (50 q8h)	25-50 q6h	1-2 q4-q12h	1 g 40 2 g 80-90	≤8
Ceftriaxone (IV, IM)	50 q24h (50 q24h)	50-80 q24h (50 q24h)	50 q24h CNS: 80 q24h	0.5-2 q24h	1 g 150 1 g 50	≤8
Ceftazidime (IV, IM)	30 q8h (50 q12h)	50 q8h (50 q8h)	25-50 q6h	0.5-2 q8-12h	1 g 85 1 g 34	
Amikacin (IV, IM)	10 q12h (7.5 q12h)	10 q8h (7.5 q8h)	5 q8h or 7.5 q12h	5 mg/kg q8h or 7.5 mg/kg q12h	20-40 20	≤16
Gentamicin (IV, IM)	2.5 q12h (2.5 q12h)	2.5 q8h (2.5 q8h)	1-2.5 q8h	1-1.7 mg/kg q8h	4-10 7	≤4
Tobramycin (IV, IM)	2 q12h (2 q12h)	2 q8h (2 q8h)	1-2 q8h	1-1.7 mg/kg q8h	4-14 4	≤4

Trimethoprim-sulfamethoxazole (TMP-SMX) (PO, IV)	Not recommended	Not recommended	3-6 TMP/15-30 SMX q12h / 5 TMP/25 SMX q6h for pneumocystosis	0.16 TMP/0.8 SMX q12h	2-4/80-100	≤2/38
Sulfisoxazole (PO)	Not recommended	Not recommended	30-37.5 q6h	0.5-1 q6h	40-50	≤100 (urinary tract infection only)
Erythromycin estolate (PO)	10 q12h (10 q12h)	10-12.5 q8h (10 q8h)	10 q8h or 15 q12h	0.25-0.5 q6h	4.2	≤0.5
Erythromycin ethylsuccinate (PO)	10 q12h (10 q12h)	10 q8h (10 q8h)	10 q6h	0.25-0.5 q6h	1.5	≤0.5
Clindamycin (PO, IV)	5 q8h (5 q12h)	5 q6h (5 q8h)	2.5-7.5 q6h	0.15-0.45 q6h	2.5-3.6	≤0.5
Chloramphenicol (IV, PO)	25 q24h (25 q24h)	25 q24h (25 q24h)	12.5-18.75 q6h / 18.75-25 q6h (meningitis)	12.5-25 **mg/kg** q6h	19 / 25	*H. influenzae* ≤4 / Others ≤12.5
Tetracycline (IV, PO)	Not recommended	Not recommended	Children >8 yr 6.25-12.5 q6h	0.25-0.5 q6h	8 / 4	≤4
Vancomycin (IV)	15 q12h (10 q12h)	10 q8h (10 q8h)	10-15 q6h	15 **mg/kg** q12h or 6.25-8 **mg/kg** q6h	30-40	≤5
Metronidazole (PO, IV)	7.5 q12h (7.5 q12h)	7.5 q12h (7.5 q12h)	5-12 q8h / 7.5 q6h	7.5 **mg/kg** q6h	11.5 / 20-25	≤4
Rifampin (PO)	Not recommended	Not recommended	10-20 q24h	0.6 q24h	7	≤1

See *Primary Pediatric Care*, ed 3, p. 377.

Antimicrobials, peak serum concentrations

Times that peak serum concentrations are reached after administration of antimicrobial agents

	Route of administration	Time of peak concentration*
Penicillins	IV	5 min
Cephalosporins	IV	5 min
Penicillin V	PO	30 min - 1 hr
Amoxicillin	PO	2 hr
Cephalexin	PO	1 hr
Aminoglycosides	IV	30 min
	IM	1 hr
Trimethoprim-sulfamethoxazole	PO	1-2 hr
Sulfisoxazole	PO	2-3 hr
Erythromycin (estolate or ethylsuccinate)	PO	2 hr
Clindamycin	PO	1-2 hr
Chloramphenicol	PO/IV	2 hr
Vancomycin	IV	2 hr
Rifampin	PO	2 hr

*For drugs given intravenously, the time of peak serum concentrations is stated in minutes or hours after *completion* of the infusion.

IV, Intravenous; *PO*, oral; *IM*, intramuscular.

See *Primary Pediatric Care*, ed 3, p. 374.

Antiviral drugs

Generic (trade name)	Indication		Normal recommended dosage
Acyclovir* (Zovirax)	Genital herpes simplex virus (HSV) infection, first episode	PO	1200 mg/day in 3 divided doses for 7-10 days†
	Genital HSV infection, recurrence	IV	15 mg/kg/day in 3 divided doses for 5-7 days
	Recurrent genital HSV episodes in patient with frequent recurrences:	PO	1200 mg/day in 3 divided doses or 1600 mg/day in 2 divided doses for 5 days†
	Chronic suppressive therapy	PO	800-1000 mg/day in 2-5 divided doses for as long as 12 continuous months†
	HSV in immunocompromised host (localized, progressive, or disseminated)‡	IV	*Children <1 yr except neonates:* 15-30 mg/kg/day in 3 divided doses for 7-14 days (some experts also recommend this dosage for children ≥1 yr)
		IV	*Children ≥1 yr:* 750 mg/m²/day in 3 divided doses for 7-14 days (some experts recommend 1500 mg/m²/day in 3 divided doses)
	Prophylaxis of HSV in immunocompromised HSV-seropositive patient‡	PO	1000 mg/day in 3-5 divided doses for 7-14 days†
		PO	600-1000 mg/day in 3-5 divided doses during risk period†
		IV	750 mg/m²/day in 3 divided doses during risk period
	HSV encephalitis	IV	*Children <1 yr:* 30 mg/kg/day in 3 divided doses for a minimum of 14 days (some experts also recommend this dosage for children ≥1 yr)
		IV	*Children ≥1 yr:* 1500 mg/m²/day in 3 divided doses for 14-21 days (some experts also recommend this dosage for children <1 yr)
	Neonatal HSV‡	IV	30 mg/kg/day in 3 divided doses for 14-21 days (some experts recommend 45-60 mg/kg/day in 3 divided doses for term infants; for premature infants, 20 mg/kg/day in 2 divided doses is recommended for 14-21 days)

Continued.

See *Primary Pediatric Care,* ed 3, p. 392.

Antiviral drugs

Generic (trade name)	Indication		Normal recommended dosage
Acyclovir* (Zovirax)	Varicella or zoster in immuno-compromised host	IV	*Children <1 yr:* 30 mg/kg/day in 3 divided doses (some experts also recommend this dosage for children ≥1 yr)
			Children ≥1 yr: 1500 mg/m²/day in 3 divided doses for 7-10 days
	Zoster in immunocompetent host‡	IV	Same as for zoster in immunocompromised host
		PO	4000 mg/day in 5 divided doses for 5-7 days for patients ≥12 yr†
	Varicella in immunocompetent host	PO	80 mg/kg/day in 4 divided doses for 5 days; maximum dose is 3200 mg/day
	Prophylaxis of cytomegalovirus (CMV) infection in immuno-compromised host (e.g., trans-plant recipient)‡	PO	800-3200 mg/day in 1-4 divided doses during risk period*†
		IV	1500 mg/m²/day in 3 divided doses during risk period
Amantadine (Symmetrel)	Influenza A: treatment and pro-phylaxis	PO >20 kg:	100 mg/day in 1 or 2 divided doses for duration of exposure
		<20 kg:	5 mg/kg/day in 1 or 2 divided doses for duration of exposure
Ribavirin (Virazole)	Treatment of respiratory syncytial virus (RSV) infection	Aerosol	Given by a small particle generator, in a solution of 6 g in 300 ml of sterile water (20 mg/ml), for 12-20 hours/day for 1-7 days; longer treatment may be necessary for some patients
Rimantadine (Flumadine)	Influenza A: treatment and pro-phylaxis	PO >20 kg:	100 mg/day in 1 or 2 divided doses for duration of exposure
		<20 kg:	5 mg/kg/day in 1 or 2 divided doses for duration of exposure
Vidarabine (Vira-A)	Neonatal HSV	IV	15-30 mg/kg/day in 1 dose over 12-24 hr for 10-21 days
	Varicella or zoster in immuno-compromised host‡	IV	10 mg/kg/day in 1 dose over 12-24 hr for 5-10 days

Modified from Peter G et al, editors: Report of the Committee on Infectious Diseases: *1994 Red Book,* ed 23, Elk Grove Village, Ill, 1994, The American Academy of Pediatrics.

*Dose should be reduced if the patient's renal function is impaired.

†In children, oral dose of acyclovir should not exceed 80 mg/day.

‡As of June 1994 the drug had not been licensed for this use or was investigational.

Use and complications of chemotherapeutic agents in acute leukemia

Drug (route)	Common use	Acute toxicity	Delayed toxic effects
Prednisone (PO)	Induction and maintenance of ALL	Hyperglycemia, hypertension, emotional lability, increased appetite, fluid retention, weight gain, striae, cushingoid facies, peptic ulcer, diabetes mellitus	Osteoporosis, growth retardation, aseptic necrosis, cataracts, glaucoma, diabetes mellitus
Vincristine (IV)	Induction and maintenance of ALL	Alopecia, constipation, paralytic ileus, peripheral neuropathy, jaw pain, SIADH,* danger with extravasation, in rare cases, myelosuppression	Peripheral neuropathy
6-Mercaptopurine (PO, IV)	Maintenance of ALL	Alopecia, nausea, vomiting, diarrhea, myelosuppression, hepatic damage, cholestasis	Hepatic disease, cholestasis
Methotrexate (PO, IM, IV)	Maintenance of ALL	Nausea, vomiting, mucositis, rash, myelosuppression, hepatic damage, renal toxicity	Hepatic damage, neurotoxicity
Methotrexate and/or cytosine arabinoside (Intrathecal)	CNS prophylaxis of ALL and ANLL	Nausea, vomiting, headache, stiff neck, arachnoiditis, seizures	Cortical atrophy, leukoencephalopathy
L-Asparaginase (IM)	Induction and consolidation of ALL	Anaphylaxis, nausea, vomiting, fever, chills, hyperglycemia, diabetes, abdominal pain, pancreatitis (increased amylase), CNS depression, coagulation defects with thrombosis or hemorrhage (i.e., stroke), hypoproteinemia, hepatic damage	Pancreatic or hepatic damage, diabetes mellitus
Doxorubicin (IV)	Induction and consolidation of ALL	Myelosuppression, alopecia, nausea, vomiting, mucositis, anorexia, hepatic damage, cardiac arrhythmias, red urine, danger with extravasation	Cardiomyopathy, hepatic damage

Continued.

Chemotherapeutic agents, acute leukemia—cont'd

Use and complications of chemotherapeutic agents in acute leukemia—cont'd

Drug (route)	Common use	Acute toxicity	Delayed toxic effects
Daunorubicin (IV)	Induction and maintenance of ALL and ANLL	Myelosuppression, alopecia, nausea, vomiting, cardiac arrhythmias, hepatic damage, red urine, danger with extravasation	Cardiomyopathy
Cytosine arabinoside (IV)	Induction and maintenance of ANLL	Myelosuppression, alopecia, nausea, vomiting, diarrhea, mucositis, conjunctivitis, fever, neurotoxicity	Hepatic damage, neurotoxicity
	Consolidation of high-risk ALL		
Etoposide/tenoposide (IV)	Induction and maintenance of ANLL	Hypotension, anaphylaxis, myelosuppression, nausea, vomiting, alopecia, mucositis, danger with extravasation	Second malignancy, most commonly ANLL
	Consolidation of high-risk ALL		
6-Thioguanine (PO)	Induction and maintenance of ANLL	Same as for mercaptopurine but less hepatic toxicity	
Radiation	ALL	Alopecia, nausea, vomiting, skin hypersensitivity, mild myelosuppression	Sleeping syndrome, seizures, leukoencephalopathy, growth retardation
	CNS prophylaxis		

Data compiled from Dorr RT, Fritz WL: *Cancer chemotherapy handbook*. New York, 1980, Elsevier.
*SIADH, Syndrome of inappropriate secretion of antidiuretic hormone.

See *Primary Pediatric Care*, ed 3, p. 1405.

Products for coagulation disorders

Product	Content	Dose or concentration	Indications/comments
Fresh-frozen plasma	200-240 ml whole plasma	5-15 ml/kg; 1 U factor/ml	Contains all plasma factors; for multiple factor deficiency, DIC, reversal of coumadin effect, HUS, or TTP, unknown coagulation defect; not virus inactivated
Cryoprecipitate	Factor VIII, VWF, factor XIII, fibrinogen, fibronectin	± 75-100 U factor VIII or VWF/bag; volume ±20 ml	From single donor units; not virus inactivated
Prothrombin complex	Factors II, VII, IX, and X	Preassayed for factor IX; factor VII content varies among products (high and assayed in Proplex); dose for inhibitor 100-150 u/kg	Hemophilia B; mild bleeding in hemophilia A with inhibitor; congenital deficiency of factor II, VII, or X; danger of thrombosis (including MI and DIC) with liver disease, vascular disease, prolonged use; virus inactivated*
Factor VIII	Factor VIII; VWF in Humate P	Preassayed; up to 100 u/ml	Hemophilia A; Humate P for VWD†; recombinant product available; virus inactivated; DDAVP is preferred for type I VWD and mild hemophilia when possible
Factor IX	Factor IX	Preassayed	Hemophilia B; virus inactivated*
Activated prothrombin complex	Factors II, VII, IX, and X; factor VIII "bypassing" activity	50-100 u/kg up to q6-8h	Cannot evaluate response by measuring factor VIII activity; risk of thrombosis
Hyate:C	Porcine factor VIII	Preassayed	Hemophilia A with inhibitor that is not cross-reactive

*Virus attenuation processes may not inactivate parvovirus, hepatitis A, and possibly other viruses.
†Has not been approved by the FDA for use in VWD.
DDAVP, Desmopressin; *DIC*, disseminated intravascular coagulation; *MI*, myocardial infarction; *VWD*, von Willebrand disease; *VWF*, von Willebrand factor.

See *Primary Pediatric Care*, ed 3, p. 359.

Medications for constipation and impaction

Medication	Dosage	Comments
Stool softeners		
Mineral oil	1-2 ml/kg/dose bid Adolescents: 60 ml/dose (max 8 oz/day)	Do not use in children who have GE reflux or vomiting or who are not yet walking Emulsified types (Petrogalar, plain Agoral, Kondremul) taste better
Lactulose	0.5-1.0 ml/kg/dose bid Adolescents: 15 ml bid (max 3 oz/day)	Prescription item
Laxatives*		
Phillips' Milk of Magnesia or Haley's M-O (75% MOM, 25% mineral oil)	1 ml/kg/dose bid Adolescents: 60 ml bid	1 tab MOM = 2.5 ml liquid
Senokot	<5 yr: 1-2 tsp syrup >5 yr: 2-3 tsp syrup Adolescents: 1 tbsp (max 2.5 tbsp or 8 tabs)	1 tab = 3 ml granules = 5 ml syrup
Fletcher's Castoria	<5 yr: 1-2 tsp >5 yr: 2-3 tsp Adolescents: 2 tbsp max	
Dulcolax, 5-mg tab	>5 yr: 5 mg >12 yr: 10 mg (2 tabs) Adolescents: 4 tabs max	No liquid form
Phenolphthalein	>5 years: ½ tab Adolescents: 1 tab	Chewable tabs (Ex-Lax) 90 mg
Rectal suppositories		
Glycerin suppository	1 or 2	
Dulcolax, 10 mg	>2 yr: 1 suppository	
Enemas		
Mineral oil enema	1-2 oz/20 lb of weight Adolescents: 4 oz	Squeeze-bottle size: 4.5 oz
Sodium phosphate enema (Fleet)	1 oz/20 lb of weight Adolescents: 4 oz (max 8 oz)	Squeeze-bottle size: 2.25 oz children, 4.5 oz adult

Modified from Schmitt BD, Mauro RD: *Contemp Pediatr* 9:47, 1992.
*Listed in order of increasing potency.

See *Primary Pediatric Care,* ed 3, p. 723.

Drugs commonly used to treat neonatal drug abstinence syndrome

Drugs	Dosage
Paregoric	3-6 drops q4-6h PO
Laudanum (0.4%)	3-6 drops q4-6h PO
Chlorpromazine	2-3 mg/kg/day q6h PO
Phenobarbital	3-6 mg/kg/day q6h PO

See *Primary Pediatric Care,* ed 3, p. 565.

Neonatal drug
abstinence syndrome

Nonsteroidal antiinflammatory drugs

Dosage guidelines for commonly used nonsteroidal antiinflammatory drugs (NSAIDs)

Generic name	Brand name	Dose (mg/kg) frequency	Maximum adult daily dose (mg)	Comments
Salicylates (aspirin)	Bayer, Bufferin, Anacin, Alka-Seltzer, others	10-15 q 4 hr	4000	Inhibits platelet aggregation, GI irritability, Reye syndrome
Acetaminophen	Tylenol, "aspirin-free," Panadol, Tempra, others	10-15 q 4 hr	4000	Lacks antiinflammatory activity
Ibuprofen	Motrin, Advil, Medipren, others	6-10 q 6-8 hr	2400	Available as an oral suspension
Naproxen	Naprosyn	5-10 q 12 hr	1000	Available as an oral suspension
Indomethacin	Indocin	0.3-1 q 6 hr	150	Commonly used in NICU to close patent ductus arteriosus
Ketorolac	Toradol	IV or IM: Load 0.5, maintenance 0.2-0.5 q 6 hr	150	May be given orally; Adult IM dosing: Load 30 mg, followed by 15-30 mg q 6 hr
Choline-magnesium trisalicylate	Trilisate	8-10 q 8-12 hr	4000	Does not bind to platelets; see Salicylate

See *Primary Pediatric Care*, ed 3, p. 1528.

Drugs used in pediatric advanced life support

Drug	Dose	Comments
Adenosine	0.1-0.2 mg/kg (max: 12 mg in a single dose)	Rapid IV bolus
Atropine sulfate	0.02 mg/kg/dose	Dose may be repeated once
	Minimum dose: 0.1 mg	
	Maximum single dose:	
	Child: 0.5 mg	
	Adolescent: 1 mg	
Bretylium	5 mg/kg; may be increased to 10 mg/kg	Rapid IV bolus
Calcium chloride 10%	20 mg/kg/dose; repeat in 10 min if necessary	Administer slowly
(100 mg/ml)		Not for cardiac arrest
		Use for hypocalcemia, hypermagnesemia, and channel blocker
		Overdose
Dobutamine HCl	2-20 μg/kg/min	Titrate to desired effect
Dopamine HCl	2-20 μg/kg/min	Titrate to desired effect
Epinephrine		
For bradycardia	*IV/IO:* 0.01 mg/kg	Be aware of preservative administered when large doses are used
	(0.1 ml/kg)	
	1:10,000	
	ET: 0.1 mg/kg	
	(0.1 ml/kg)	
	1:1000	
For asystole or pulse-	**First dose:**	Be aware of preservative administered when large doses are used
less arrest	*IV/IO:* 0.01 mg/kg	
	1:10,000	

Continued.

Pediatric advanced life support drugs

Drugs used in pediatric advanced life support—cont'd

Drug	Dose	Comments
Epinephrine—cont'd	*ET:* 0.1 mg/kg	
	1:1000 class IIb*	
	Doses as high as 0.2 mg/kg may be effective	
	Subsequent doses:	
	IV/IO/ET: 0.1 mg/kg	
	1:1000 class IIa*	
	Doses as high as 0.2 mg/kg may be effective, class IIa	Repeat q3-5 min
Epinephrine infusion	*Initial:* 0.1 µg/kg/min	Titrate to desired effect 0.1-1 µg/kg/min
	Use higher infusion dose with asystole: 20 µg/kg/min	Lower dose with effective pulses
Lidocaine	1 mg/kg/dose	
Lidocaine infusion	20-50 µg/kg/min	Infuse slowly and only if ventilation is adequate
Sodium bicarbonate	1 mEq/kg/dose	Not for cardiac arrest
	or	Use for metabolic acidosis
	0.3 × kg × base deficit	
	Subsequent doses are based on blood gas analysis every 10 min of arrest	

From the Emergency Cardiac Care Committee and Subcommittees of the American Heart Association, *JAMA* 268:2662, 1992.
*Based on classification on supporting scientific evidence.
ET, Endotracheal; *IO,* intraosseous; *IV,* intravenous.

See *Primary Pediatric Care,* ed 3, p. 1791.

Red blood cell preparations

Product	Preparation	Hematocrit (%) or cell count	Volume/unit (ml)	Indications/comments
Whole blood	450 ml blood, plus anticoagulant	40%	500	Massive bleeding, exchange transfusion
Packed RBCs	Centrifuged or sedimented to remove about two thirds of plasma	80%	250	Most RBC transfusions
Buffy coat–depleted RBCs	Centrifuged to remove white cell layer	90% Contains 15%–30% of original WBCs	200	Chronically transfused patients; patients who have severe febrile reactions
Washed RBCs	Several manual and automated techniques available to remove plasma; must be used within 24 hours	90% Contains <1% of original plasma, <10% of WBCs	200	Repeated febrile and allergic reactions
Frozen RBCs	Frozen in glycerol, thawed, and washed; must be used within 24 hours of thawing; 10%–15% loss of original RBCs	Contains <0.025% of original plasma, 1%–5% of original WBCs and platelets	200	Rare blood types, multiple severe febrile/allergic reactions, IgA deficiency, autologous blood donations

See *Primary Pediatric Care,* ed 3, p. 356.

Resuscitation medications, neonatal

Medications for neonatal resuscitation

Medication	Concentration to administer	Preparation (ml)	Dosage/route*	Weight (kg)	Total dose/infant Total ml	Rate/precautions
Epinephrine	1:10,000	1	0.1-0.3 ml/kg	1	0.1-0.3	Give rapidly
				2	0.2-0.6	
				3	0.3-0.9	
			IV or IT	4	0.4-1.2	
Volume expanders	Whole blood 5% Albumin Normal saline Lactated Ringer	40	10 ml/kg IV	1	10	Give over 5-10 min
				2	20	
				3	30	
				4	40	
				Weight (kg)	**Total dose (mEq)** **Total ml**	
Sodium bicarbonate	0.5 mEq/mL (4.2% solution)	20 or two 10 prefilled syringes	2 mEq/kg IV	1	2 4	Give *slowly*, over at least 2 min
				2	4 8	Give only if infant being effectively ventilated
				3	6 12	
				4	8 16	

From American Academy of Pediatrics: *Textbook of neonatal resuscitation*, Dallas, 1990, American Heart Association.

*_IM_, Intramuscular; _IT_, intratracheal; _IV_, intravenous; _SQ_, subcutaneous.

Naloxone	0.4 mg/ml	1	0.25 ml/kg		Total ml	
				1	0.25	
			IV, IM, SQ, IT	2	0.50	
				3	0.75	
				4	1.00	
	1.0 mg/ml	1	0.1 ml/kg	1	0.1	
				2	0.2	
			IV, IM, SQ, IT	3	0.3	Give rapidly
				4	0.4	

Dopamine	$\dfrac{\text{weight}}{6 \times (\text{kg})} \times \dfrac{\text{desired dose}}{(\mu g/kg/min)}$	Begin at 5 μg/kg/min (may increase to 20 μg/kg/min if necessary) IV		Total μg/min	
	$\dfrac{}{\text{desired fluid (ml/hr)}}$		1	5-20	Give as a continuous infusion using an infusion pump
	$= \text{per 100 ml of}$		2	10-40	Monitor HR and BP closely
	solution		3	15-60	Seek consultation
			4	20-80	

See *Primary Pediatric Care*, ed 3, p. 556.

Stimulant medication, attention deficit/hyperactivity disorder

Guidelines for use of stimulant medication in children who have AD/HD

Medication	Starting amount per dose	Suggested increments	Doses/day	Time of administration
Methylphenidate (Ritalin)	0.3 mg/kg*	0.15 mg/kg	2-3	8 AM, noon, 4 PM
Methylphenidate, sustained release (Ritalin-SR)†	20 mg	20 mg	1	8 AM
Dextroamphetamine (Dexedrine)				
Tablets	0.15 mg/kg*	0.08 mg/kg	2-3	8 AM, noon, 4 PM
	≤7 yr: 5 mg	5 mg	1	8 AM
	≥8 yr: 10 mg	5 mg	1	8 AM
Spansules	≤7 yr: 37.5 mg	18.75 mg	1‡	8 AM
	≥8 yr: 75 mg	37.5 mg	1	8 AM
Pemoline (Cylert)				

*Suggested starting dose of methylphenidate and dextroamphetamine (mg/kg) refers to the *amount per dose*; the amount per day is greater, depending on the frequency of administration.
†The sustained-release form of methylphenidate is available only in a 20 mg size. If the child's total daily dose is close to 20 mg, this form may be used.
‡Some physicians give an additional dose at 4 PM: 18.75 mg for younger children and 37.5 mg for older children.

See *Primary Pediatric Care*, ed 3, p. 676.

Drugs used commonly for the treatment of tuberculosis among infants, children, and adolescents

Drugs	Dosage form	Daily dose (mg/kg/day)	Dose (mg/kg/dose) Twice weekly	Maximum dose Twice weekly	Adverse reactions
Ethambutol	Tablets 100 mg 400 mg	15-25	50	2.5 g	Optic neuritis (reversible), diminished visual acuity, reduced red-green color discrimination, GI disturbance
Isoniazid*	Scored tablets 100 mg 300 mg Syrup 10 mg/ml	10-15	20-30	Daily: 300 mg; twice weekly: 900 mg	Mild hepatic enzyme elevation, hepatitis, peripheral neuritis, hypersensitivity
Pyrazinamide*	Scored tablets 500 mg	20-40	50	2 g	Hepatotoxicity, hyperuricemia
Rifampin*	Capsules 150 mg 300 mg Syrup (formulated in syrup from capsules)	10-20	10-20	600 mg	Orange discoloration of secretions/urine, staining of contact lenses, hepatitis, flulike reaction, thrombocytopenia; may render birth control pills ineffective
Streptomycin (intramuscular administration)	Vials 1 g 4 g	20-40	20-40	1 g	Ototoxicity, nephrotoxicity, skin rash

*Rifamate is a capsule containing 150 mg of isoniazid and 300 mg of rifampin. Rifater is a tablet containing 50 mg of isoniazid, 120 mg of rifampin, and 300 mg of pyrazinamide.

See *Primary Pediatric Care*, ed 3, p. 1634.

Specific vasopressor agents used to treat shock

Agent	Site of action (receptor)	Dose* (µg/kg/min)	Effect
Dopamine	δ	1-3	"Dopaminergic;" renal vasodilation; inotropic
	α>β	5-20	Peripheral vasoconstriction; increased systemic vascular resistance; dysrhythmias
Dobutamine	β₁, β₂	1-20	Inotropic, chronotropic; vasodilation (β₂); lowers systemic vascular resistance; lowers pulmonary vascular resistance; tachycardia and arrhythmia (β₁)
Epinephrine	α>β	0.05-1.0	Inotropic
			Tachycardia; arrhythmia; decreased renal flow from α effect; increase in myocardial oxygen consumption; intense vasoconstriction
Norepinephrine	α>β	0.005-1.0	Profound vasoconstriction; inotropic; dramatic increase in myocardial oxygen consumption and systemic vascular resistance

*The doses listed are suggested starting ranges. The drugs can be titrated to the desired effect depending on the patient's response.

See *Primary Pediatric Care*, ed 3, p. 1767.

White cell and platelet preparations

Product	Preparation	Cell count	Volume/unit (ml)	Indications/comments
Random donor platelets	Separated from single whole blood units	$5-7 \times 10^{10}$ platelets/unit	50	Infants, short-term need; 1 unit/10 kg increases platelet count by 50,000
Single donor platelets	Collected by apheresis	Equivalent to 6-10 random units	200-400 usually in two bags	Patients who require repeated transfusions
Buffy coat granulocytes	Separated from single whole blood units	$0.35-5 \times 10^9$/unit	25	? usefulness; must be ABO-compatible; must be used within 24 hours of collection
Apheresed granulocyte concentrates	Various techniques to increase donor neutrophil count and yield	$0.5-3 \times 10^{10}$/unit	500	Contains RBCs, must be ABO-compatible; must be used within 24 hours of collection

See *Primary Pediatric Care*, ed 3, p. 358.

Miscellaneous Information

Laboratory parameters of acid-base disturbances*

	pH	Arterial carbon dioxide pressure (PaCO₂)	Bicarbonate (HCO₃⁻) (mEq/L)	Carbon dioxide (CO₂) content (mEq/L)
Normal values	7.35-7.45	35-45	24-26	25-28
Disturbances				
Metabolic acidosis	↓	↓	↓	↓
Acute respiratory acidosis	↓	↑	↕	Slight ↑
Compensated respiratory acidosis	↔ or slight↓	↑	↑	↑
Metabolic alkalosis	↑	Slight ↑	↑	↑
Acute respiratory alkalosis	↑	↓	↕	Slight ↓
Compensated respiratory alkalosis	↔ or slight ↑	↓	↓	↓

*Values obtained by arteriolized capillary blood or direct arterial puncture.

See *Primary Pediatric Care*, ed 3, p. 1821.

Adolescent development

Order of adolescent development

Male

Enlargement of testes
Pubic hair
Axillary hair
Facial hair

Female

Growth acceleration
Breast development
Pubic hair
Menarche
Axillary hair

See *Primary Pediatric Care,* ed 3, p. 951.

Airway obstruction

Scoring system for assessing the severity of upper airway obstruction

Sign	Score*
Stridor	
None	0
Inspiratory	1
Inspiratory and expiratory	2
Cough	
None	0
Hoarse cry	1
Bark	2
Retractions and nasal flaring	
None	0
Flaring and suprasternal retractions	1
Flaring plus suprasternal, subcostal, and intercostal retractions	2
Cyanosis	
None	0
In room air	1
In 40% oxygen	2
Inspiratory breath sounds	
Normal	0
Harsh, with wheezing or ronchi	1
Delayed	2

From Downes JJ, Goldberg AI: Airway management, mechanical ventilation, and cardiopulmonary resuscitation. In Scarpelli EM, Auld PAM, Goldman HS, editors: *Pulmonary disease of the fetus, newborn, and child,* Philadelphia, 1978, Lea & Febiger.
*A score of 4 or higher indicates significant airway obstruction.

See *Primary Pediatric Care,* ed 3, p. 1651.

Topics of anticipatory guidance

Prenatal and newborn
Prenatal visit
1. *Health:* pregnancy course; worries; tobacco, alcohol, drug use; hospital and pediatric office procedures
2. *Safety:* infant car seat, crib safety
3. *Nutrition:* planned feeding method
4. *Child care:* help after birth, later arrangements
5. *Family:* changes in relationships (spouse, siblings), supports, stresses, return to work

Newborn visits
1. *Health:* jaundice, umbilical cord care, circumcision, other common problems, when to call pediatrician's office
2. *Safety:* infant car seat, smoke detector, choking, keeping tap water temperature below 120° F
3. *Nutrition:* feeding, normal weight loss, spitting, vitamin and fluoride supplements
4. *Development/behavior:* individuality, "consolability," visual and auditory responsiveness
5. *Child care:* importance of interaction, parenting books, support for primary caregiver
6. *Family:* postpartum adjustments, fatigue, "blues," special time for siblings

First year
Up to 6 months
1. *Health:* immunizations, exposure to infections
2. *Safety:* falls, aspiration of small objects or powder, entanglement in mobiles that have long strings
3. *Nutrition:* supplementing breast milk or formula, introducing solids, iron
4. *Development/behavior:* crying/colic, irregular schedules (eating, sleeping, eliminating), response to infant cues, reciprocity, interactive games, beginning eye-hand coordination
5. *Child care:* responsive and affectionate care, caregiving schedule
6. *Family:* return to work, nurturing of all family relationships (spouse and siblings)

6 to 12 months
1. *Safety:* locks for household poisons and medications; gates for stairs; ipecac; poison center telephone number; outlet safety covers; avoiding dangling cords or tablecloths; safety devices for windows/screens; toddler car seat when infant reaches 20 pounds; avoiding toys that have small detachable pieces; supervise child in tub or near water
2. *Nutrition:* discouraging use of bottle as a pacifier or while in bed; offering cup and soft finger foods (with supervision); introducing new foods one at a time
3. *Development/behavior:* attachment, basic trust versus mistrust, stranger awareness, night waking, separation anxiety, bedtime routine, transitional object
4. *Child care:* prohibitions few but firm and consistent across caregiving settings; defining discipline as "learning" (not punishment)
5. *Family:* spacing of children

See *Primary Pediatric Care,* ed 3, p. 151.

Continued

Topics of anticipatory guidance—cont'd

Second year

1 to 2 years

1. *Health:* immunizations
2. *Safety:* climbing and falls common; supervising outdoor play; ensuring safety caps on medicine bottles; noting dangers of plastic bags, pan handles hanging over stove, and space heaters
3. *Nutrition:* avoiding feeding conflicts (decreased appetite is common); period of self-feeding, weaning from breast or bottle; avoiding sweet or salty snacks
4. *Development/behavior:* autonomy versus shame/doubt, ambivalence (independence/dependence), tantrums, negativism, getting into everything, night fears, readiness for toilet training, self-comforting behaviors (thumb sucking, masturbation), speech, imaginative play, no sharing in play, positive reinforcement for desired behavior
5. *Child care:* freedom to explore in safe place; day care; home a safer place to vent frustrations; needs show of affection, language stimulation through reading and conversation
6. *Family:* sibling relationships, parents modeling of nonaggressive responses to conflict (including their own conflict with their toddler)

Preschool

2 to 5 years

1. *Health:* tooth brushing, first dental visit
2. *Safety:* needs close supervision near water or street; home safety factors include padding of sharp furniture corners, fire escape plan for home, and locking up power tools; should have car lap belt at 40 pounds and bike helmet; should know (a) name, address, and telephone number, (b) not to provoke dogs, and (c) to say "no" to strangers
3. *Nutrition:* balanced diet; avoiding sweet or salty snacks; participating in conversation at meals
4. *Development/behavior:* initiative versus guilt; difficulty with impulse control and sharing; developing interest in peers; high activity level; speaking in sentences by age 3; speech mostly intelligible to stranger by age 3; reading books; curiosity about body parts; magical thinking; egocentrism
5. *Child care/preschool:* needs daily special time with parents, bedtime routine; talking about day in day care; limiting TV watching with child; reprimanding privately; answering questions factually and simply; adjusting to preschool, kindergarten readiness
6. *Family:* chores, responsibilities

Topics of anticipatory guidance—cont'd

Middle childhood

5 to 10 years

1. *Health:* appropriate weight; regular exercise; somatic complaints (limb and abdominal pain, headaches); alcohol, tobacco, and drug use; sexual development; physician and child dealings (more direct)
2. *Safety:* bike helmets and street safety; car seat belts; swimming lessons; use of matches, firearms, and power tools; fire escape plan for home; saying "no" to strangers
3. *Nutrition:* balanced diet, daily breakfast, limiting sweet and salty snacks, moderate intake of fatty foods
4. *Development/behavior:* industry versus inferiority, need for successes, peer interactions, adequate sleep
5. *School:* school performance, homework, parent interest
6. *Family:* more time away but continuing need for family support, approval, affection, time together, and communication; family rules about bedtime, chores, and responsibilities; guidance in using money; parents should encourage reading; limiting TV watching and discussing programs seen together; teaching and modeling nonviolent responses to conflict
7. *Other activities:* organized sports, religious groups, other organizations, use of spare time

Adolescence

Discuss with adolescent

1. *Health:* alcohol, tobacco, and drug use, health consequences of violence, dental care, physical activity, immunizations
2. *Safety:* bike and skateboard helmet and safety, car seat belts, driving while intoxicated, water safety, hitchhiking, risk taking
3. *Nutrition:* balanced diet, appropriate weight, avoiding junk foods
4. *Sexuality:* physical changes, sex education, peer pressure for sexual activity, sense of responsibility for self and partner, OK to say no, preventing pregnancy and sexually transmitted diseases, breast and testes self-examination
5. *Development/relationships:* identity versus role confusion, family, peers, dating, independence, trying different roles, managing anger other than with verbal and physical attacks
6. *School:* academics, homework
7. *Other activities:* sports, hobbies, organizations, jobs
8. *Future plans:* school, work, relationships with others

Discuss with parents

1. *Communication:* allowing adolescents to participate in discussion and development of family rules; needs frequent praise and affection, time together, interest in adolescent's activities
2. *Independence:* parent and child ambivalence about independence; expecting periods of estrangement; promoting self-responsibility and independence; still needs supervision
3. *Role model:* actions speak louder than words—parents provide model of responsible, reasonable, nonviolent, and compassionate behavior

The Apgar score

Sign	Score		
	0	1	2
Heart rate	Absent	<100	>100
Respiratory effort	Absent	Weak, irregular	Good, crying
Muscle tone	Flaccid	Some flexion of extremities	Well flexed
Reflex irritability (catheter in nose)	No response	Grimace	Cough or sneeze
Color	Blue, pale	Body pink; extremities blue	Completely pink

From Klaus MH, Fanaroff AA: *Care of the high-risk neonate,* ed 4, Philadelphia, 1993, WB Saunders.

See *Primary Pediatric Care,* ed 3, p. 55.

Blood pressure in newborns

Birth weight (g)	Systolic (mm Hg)		Diastolic (mm Hg)	
	5%	95%	5%	95%
1000	35	58	16	36
1500	40	62	19	39
2000	43	67	22	41
2500	48	70	25	43
3000	50	73	28	48
3500	54	78	30	49
4000	58	81	31	51

Data from Versmold HT et al: *Pediatrics* 67:607, 1981.

See *Primary Pediatric Care,* ed 3, p. 552.

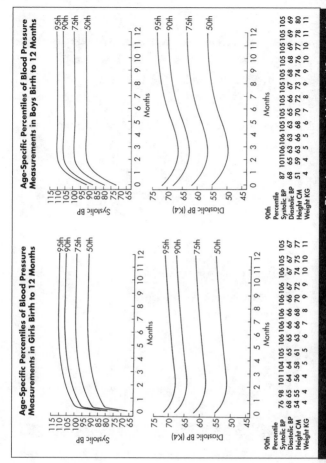

Blood pressure, birth to 12 months

Age-, gender-, height-, and weight-specific percentiles of systolic and diastolic blood pressure for birth to 12 months of age. (From Task Force on Blood Pressure Control in Children, *Pediatrics* 79:1, 1987; courtesy Dr. Michael J. Horan.)

See *Primary Pediatric Care,* ed 3, p. 1008.

Blood pressure, 1 to 13 years

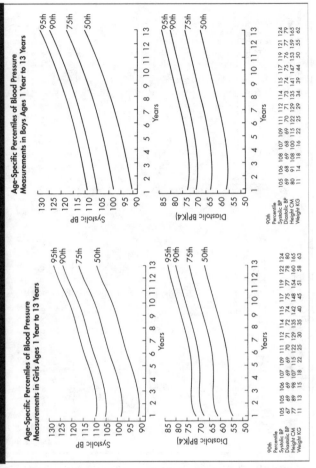

Age-, gender-, height-, and weight-specific percentiles of systolic and diastolic blood pressure for 1 to 13 years of age. (From Task Force on Blood Pressure Control in Children: *Pediatrics* 79:1, 1987; courtesy Dr. Michael J. Horan.)
See *Primary Pediatric Care,* ed 3, p. 1008.

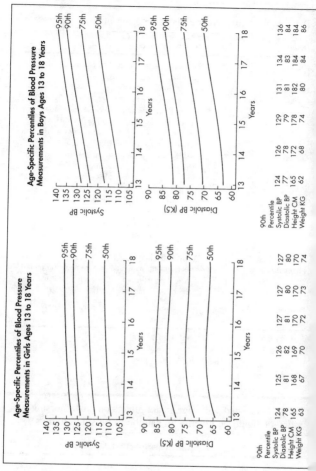

Age-, gender-, height-, and weight-specific percentiles of systolic and diastolic blood pressure for 13 to 18 years of age. (From Task Force on Blood Pressure Control in Children: *Pediatrics* 79:1, 1987; courtesy Dr Michael J. Horan.)

See *Primary Pediatric Care*, ed 3, p. 1008.

Prescription drugs contraindicated during breast-feeding

Drug	Reason for concern
Bromocriptine	Suppresses lactation; may be hazardous to the mother
Cocaine	Cocaine intoxication
Cyclophosphamide	Possible immune suppression; unknown effect on growth or association with carcinogenesis; neutropenia
Cyclosporine	Possible immune suppression; unknown effect on growth or association with carcinogenesis
Doxorubicin*	Possible immune suppression; unknown effect on growth or association with carcinogenesis
Ergotamine	Vomiting, diarrhea, convulsions (doses used in migraine medications)
Lithium	One-third to one-half therapeutic blood concentration in infants
Methotrexate	Possible immune suppression; unknown effect on growth or association with carcinogenesis; neutropenia
Phencyclidine (PCP)	Potent hallucinogen
Phenindione	Anticoagulant; increased prothrombin and partial thromboplastin time in one infant; not used in the United States

From the Committee on Drugs, American Academy of Pediatrics: *Pediatrics* 93:137, 1994.
*Drug is concentrated in human milk.

See *Primary Pediatric Care,* ed 3, p. 175.

Drugs associated with significant effects on some nursing infants (should be given with caution to nursing mothers)

Drug	Reported effect
5-Aminosalicylic acid	Diarrhea (one case)
Aspirin (salicylates)	Metabolic acidosis (one case)
Clemastine	Drowsiness, irritability, refusal to feed, high-pitched cry, neck stiffness (one case)
Phenobarbital	Sedation; infantile spasms after weaning from milk containing phenobarbital, methemoglobinemia (one case)
Primidone	Sedation, feeding problems
Sulfasalazine (salicylazosulfapyridine)	Bloody diarrhea (one case)

From the Committee on Drugs, American Academy of Pediatrics: *Pediatrics* 93:137, 1994.
When possible, the blood concentration in the infant should be measured.

See *Primary Pediatric Care,* ed 3, p. 175.

Components of human milk and infant formula

Product	Protein	Fat	Carbohydrate	Comments
Human milk	80% whey, 20% casein	Human milk fat	Lactose	
Alimentum	Hydrolized casein	50% MCT,* 40% safflower, 10% soy oils	Sucrose-modified tapioca starch	For malabsorption syndromes
Cow milk	80% casein, 20% whey	Butterfat	Lactose	
Enfamil and Enfamil with Iron	40% casein, 60% whey	55% coconut, 45% soy oils	Lactose	
Enfamil Premature	60% whey, 40% casein	40% MCT, 40% soy, 20% coconut oils	Corn syrup solids,† lactose	For premature infants
Evaporated milk base	80% casein, 20% whey	Butterfat	Lactose	Add 19 oz water and 2 tbsp. sugar to a 13 oz can of evaporated milk; supplement with multivitamins and iron
Isomil	Soy protein	60% soy, 40% coconut oils	Corn syrup solids, sucrose	For cow milk protein and/or lactose intolerance
Isomil SF	Soy protein	60% soy, 40% coconut oils	Corn syrup solids	For cow milk protein, lactose, and/or sucrose intolerance
Lofenalac	Casein hydrolysate processed to remove most of the phenylalanine	Corn oil	Corn syrup solids, modified tapioca starch	For phenylketonuria—low in phenylalanine
Nursoy‡	Soy protein	58% safflower, 27% coconut, 15% soy oils	Sucrose	For cow milk protein and/or lactose intolerance
Nutramigen	Casein hydrolysate	Corn oil	Corn syrup solids, corn starch	For sensitivity to intact milk protein or for lactose intolerance

Continued.

See *Primary Pediatric Care*, ed 3, p. 1821.

Components of human milk and infant formula—cont'd

Product	Protein	Fat	Carbohydrate	Comments
Portagen	Sodium caseinate	85% MCT; 15% corn oil	Corn syrup solids, sucrose, lactose	For fat malabsorption disorders and lactose intolerance (liver disease)
Pregestimil	Casein hydrolysate with added L-cystine, L-tyrosine, and L-tryptophan	60% MCT, 20% corn, 20% safflower oils	Corn syrup solids, dextrose, corn starch	For many malabsorption syndromes
Prosobee	Soy protein isolate	55% coconut, 45% soy oils	Corn syrup solids	For lactose and cow milk protein intolerance, sucrose intolerance, and galactosemia
RCF (Ross Carbohydrate Free)	Soy protein isolate	Coconut, soy oils	None—selected by physician	
Similac and Similac with Iron Similac PM 60/40	Nonfat cow milk 60% whey, 40% casein	60% soy, 40% coconut oils 60% coconut, 40% corn oils	Lactose Lactose	For infants predisposed to hypocalcemia (calcium/phosphorus ratio is 2:1); low salt content
Similac Special Care	60% whey, 40% casein	MCT, corn, coconut oils	Lactose, hydrolyzed corn starch	For premature infants
Similac Special Care 24	Nonfat cow milk, whey	50% MCT, coconut, soy oils	Lactose, hydrolyzed corn starch	Can be used for premature infants with fluid intolerance
SMA and SMA with Iron‡	Nonfat cow milk, demineralized whey	Oleo, oleic, coconut, soy oils	Lactose	Low salt content
SMA Preemie 24‡	60% whey, 40% casein	MCT, coconut, soy oils	Lactose, glucose	For premature infants

Modified from Johnson KB, editor: *The Harriet Lane handbook,* ed 13. Chicago, 1993, Mosby.
MCT, Medium-chain triglycerides.
†Corn syrup solids include dextrose, maltose, and other glucose polymers.
‡No longer available in the United States.

Burn Estimate Age vs Area

Area	Birth 1yr.	1-4 yr.	5-9 yr.	10-14 yr.	15 yr.	2°	3°	Total
Head	19	17	13	11	9			
Neck	2	2	2	2	2			
Ant. Trunk	13	13	13	13	13			
Post. Trunk	13	13	13	13	13			
R. Buttock	2 1/2	2 1/2	2 1/2	2 1/2	2 1/2			
L. Buttock	2 1/2	2 1/2	2 1/2	2 1/2	2 1/2			
Genitalia	1	1	1	1	1			
R.U. Arm	4	4	4	4	4			
L.U. Arm	4	4	4	4	4			
R.L. Arm	3	3	3	3	3			
L.L. Arm	3	3	3	3	3			
R. Hand	2 1/2	2 1/2	2 1/2	2 1/2	2 1/2			
L. Hand	2 1/2	2 1/2	2 1/2	2 1/2	2 1/2			
R. Thigh	5 1/2	6 1/2	8	8 1/2	9			
L. Thigh	5 1/2	6 1/2	8	8 1/2	9			
R. Leg	5	5	5 1/2	6	6 1/2			
L. Leg	5	5	5 1/2	6	6 1/2			
R. Foot	3 1/2	3 1/2	3 1/2	3 1/2	3 1/2			
L. Foot	3 1/2	3 1/2	3 1/2	3 1/2	3 1/2			
					Total			

Burn chart for estimating extent of injury. Numbers equal percentage of total body surface.
See *Primary Pediatric Care,* ed 3, p. 1777.

Triage criteria for thermal injuries

Outpatient management

Partial-thickness burn <10% body surface area (BSA)
Full-thickness burn <2% BSA

Inpatient management

Primary care hospital
Partial-thickness burn 10%-20% BSA
Full-thickness burn 2%-10% BSA
Partial-thickness burn to face, perineum, hands, or feet
Questionable burn wound depth or extent
Inadequate family support
Suspected abuse

Burn center

Partial-thickness burn >20% BSA
Full-thickness burn >10% BSA
Full-thickness burn to face, perineum, hands, or feet
Respiratory tract injury
Associated major trauma
Significant coexisting illness
Chemical or electrical burns

See *Primary Pediatric Care,* ed 3, p. 1778.

Recommended total daily calories* (moderate activity level)

Group and age (yr)	Wt (kg [lb])	Height (cm [in])	Energy needs (kcal [range])
Children			
1-3	13 (29)	90 (35)	1300 (900-1800)
4-6	20 (44)	112 (44)	1800 (1300-2300)
7-10	28 (62)	132 (52)	2000 (1650-3300)
Males			
11-14	45 (99)	157 (62)	2500 (2000-3700)
15-18	66 (145)	176 (69)	3000 (2100-3900)
19-22	70 (154)	177 (70)	2900 (2500-3300)
23-50	70 (154)	178 (70)	2900 (2300-3100)
51-75	70 (154)	178 (70)	2300 (2000-2800)
76+	70 (154)	178 (70)	2050 (1650-2450)
Females			
11-14	46 (101)	157 (62)	2200 (1500-3000)
15-18	55 (120)	163 (64)	2200 (1200-3000)
19-22	55 (120)	163 (64)	2200 (1700-2500)
23-50	55 (120)	163 (64)	2200 (1600-2400)
51-75	55 (120)	163 (64)	1900 (1400-2200)
76+	55 (120)	163 (64)	1600 (1200-2000)

Modified from the Food and Nutrition Board: *Recommended Dietary Allowances,* ed 10, Washington, DC, 1989, National Academy of Sciences, National Research Council.

*These recommendations may vary significantly up or down for specific sports and for very active children and adolescents.

See *Primary Pediatric Care,* ed 3, p. 255.

Normal ranges of cardiac function

Age (yr)	Heart rate (beats/min)	PR interval (sec)	QRS complex (sec)
<1	90-180	0.07-0.16	0.03-0.08
1-3	70-140	0.08-0.16	0.04-0.08
4-10	60-120	0.09-0.17	0.04-0.07
>10	55-110	0.09-0.20	0.04-0.08

Modified from Garson A: *Electrocardiogram in infants and children: a systematic approach,* Philadelphia, 1983, Lea & Febiger.

See *Primary Pediatric Care,* ed 3, p. 1795.

Prevalence of specific chronic conditions among children under age 18*

Condition	All	White	Black	Hispanic
Respiratory allergies	96.8	114.7	53.6	47.4
Asthma	42.5	42.0	51.3	35.1
Eczema and skin allergies	32.9	36.7	21.7	19.2
Speech defects	26.2	24.0	34.5	35.4
Digestive allergies	22.3	27.0	9.9	8.4†
Deafness and hearing loss	15.3	18.0	6.0†	15.2
Heart disease	15.2	18.3	7.7†	10.0
Musculoskeletal impairments	15.2	15.8	10.6	15.2
Blindness and vision loss	12.7	13.8	8.7†	13.3
Anemia	8.8	8.9	9.2†	7.5†
Arthritis	4.6	4.8	5.4†	2.0†
Epilepsy and seizures	2.4	1.9	2.4†	6.2†
Sickle cell disease	1.2†	<0.1†	7.1†	0.3†
Diabetes	1.0†	1.3†	<0.1†	0.3†
Other	19.8	23.6	10.2	9.2†

Adapted from Newacheck P, Stoddard J, McManus M: *Pediatrics* 91:1031, 1993.
*United States, 1988; cases per 1000.
†Prevalence estimate has a relative SE >30.

See *Primary Pediatric Care,* ed 3, p. 22.

Glasgow coma scale* modified for pediatric patients

Eye-opening response

Score	> 1 Year	< 1 Year
4	Spontaneous	Spontaneous
3	To verbal command	To shout
2	To pain	To pain
1	None	None

Motor response

Score	> 1 Year	< 1 Year
6	Obeys commands	Spontaneous response
5	Localizes pain	Localizes pain
4	Withdraws from pain	Withdraws from pain
3	Displays abnormal flexion to pain (decorticate rigidity)	Displays abnormal flexion to pain (decorticate rigidity)
2	Displays abnormal extension to pain (decerebrate rigidity)	Displays abnormal extension to pain (decerebrate rigidity)
1	None	None

Score	Verbal response		
	> 5 Years	2 to 5 Years	0-23 Months
5	Is oriented and converses	Uses appropriate words and phrases	Babbles, coos appropriately
4	Conversation is confused	Use inappropriate words	Cries, but is consolable
3	Words are inappropriate	Cries or screams persistently to pain	Cries or screams persistently to pain
2	Sounds are incomprehensible	Grunts or moans to pain	Grunts or moans to pain
1	None	None	None

Adapted from Simon J: Accidental injury and emergency medical services for children. In Behrman RE, editor: *Nelson textbook of pediatrics*, Philadelphia, 1992, WB Saunders.

*Glasgow coma score = sum of best eye opening, motor, and verbal response. Range = 3 to 15. Usual definitions of severity of head injury. Severe = score of < 9; Moderate = score of 9 to 12; Mild = score of 13 to 15.

See *Primary Pediatric Care*, ed 3, p. 1709.

Guidelines for providing a consultation

- Be precise and prompt in providing information, using language appropriate to each of the persons involved; different professionals have different jargon, but patients have variable understanding of jargon, most often none at all.
- Keep the patient and family informed but not without parallel or prior information to the referring physician.
- Be available for sharing, but not usurping, the privilege of care for a child who is referred by someone more specifically experienced in the care of adults.
- Keep thorough records and always provide the referring physician with a detailed consultation note; do not rely solely on spoken communication, whether in person or on the telephone.
- Define information with your own observations; accept the word of others only in rare circumstances.
- Be wary of "off-the-cuff" corridor or telephone consultation; when there is the least uncertainty, see the patient.

See *Primary Pediatric Care*, ed 3, p. 143.

Guidelines for requesting a consultation

- Be precise in stating your goals for the consultation and the information you need.
- Be aware of uncertainty in the patient and family and in yourself, and be prepared to take every step necessary to resolve it.
- Keep the needs of the patient and family sharply in mind, and keep them well-informed and active in the decision-making process.
- Clarify the extent to which you want only to consult or to which you want to refer and share in the care of the patient; do not abdicate your role in decision making.
- Do not abdicate your responsibilities for keeping informed, coordinating information, and maintaining continuity and communication with all the persons involved; this, of course, requires precise and detailed record keeping.

See *Primary Pediatric Care*, ed 3, p. 143.

Conversion of centimeters to inches

cm	in	cm	in
1	0.39	51	20.08
2	0.79	52	20.47
3	1.18	53	20.87
4	1.57	54	21.26
5	1.97	55	21.65
6	2.36	56	22.05
7	2.76	57	22.44
8	3.15	58	22.83
9	3.54	59	23.23
10	3.94	60	23.62
11	4.33	61	24.02
12	4.72	62	24.41
13	5.12	63	24.80
14	5.51	64	25.20
15	5.91	65	25.59
16	6.30	66	25.98
17	6.69	67	26.38
18	7.09	68	26.78
19	7.48	69	27.17
20	7.87	70	27.56
21	8.27	71	27.95
22	8.66	72	28.35
23	9.06	73	28.74
24	9.45	74	29.13
25	9.84	75	29.53
26	10.24	76	29.92
27	10.63	77	30.31
28	11.02	78	30.71
29	11.42	79	31.10
30	11.81	80	31.50
31	12.20	81	31.89
32	12.60	82	32.28
33	13.00	83	32.68
34	13.39	84	33.07
35	13.78	85	33.46
36	14.17	86	33.86
37	14.57	87	34.25
38	14.96	88	34.65
39	15.35	89	35.04
40	15.75	90	35.43
41	16.14	91	35.83
42	16.54	92	36.22
43	16.93	93	36.61
44	17.32	94	37.01
45	17.72	95	37.40
46	18.11	96	37.80
47	18.50	97	38.19
48	18.90	98	38.58
49	19.29	99	38.98
50	19.69	100	39.37

See *Primary Pediatric Care*, ed 3, p. 1821.

Continued

Conversion of centimeters to inches—cont'd

cm	in	cm	in
101	39.76	151	59.45
102	40.16	152	59.84
103	40.55	153	60.24
104	40.94	154	60.63
105	41.34	155	61.02
106	41.73	156	61.42
107	42.13	157	61.81
108	42.52	158	62.20
109	42.91	159	62.60
110	43.31	160	62.99
111	43.70	161	63.39
112	44.09	162	63.78
113	44.49	163	64.17
114	44.88	164	64.57
115	45.28	165	64.96
116	45.67	166	65.35
117	46.06	167	65.75
118	46.46	168	66.14
119	46.85	169	66.54
120	47.24	170	66.93
121	47.64	171	67.32
122	48.03	172	67.72
123	48.43	173	68.11
124	48.82	174	68.50
125	49.21	175	68.90
126	49.61	176	69.29
127	50.00	177	69.68
128	50.39	178	70.08
129	50.79	179	70.47
130	51.18	180	70.87
131	51.57	181	71.26
132	51.97	182	71.65
133	52.36	183	72.05
134	52.76	184	72.44
135	53.15	185	72.83
136	53.54	186	73.23
137	53.94	187	73.62
138	54.33	188	74.02
139	54.72	189	74.41
140	55.12	190	74.80
141	55.51	191	75.20
142	55.91	192	75.59
143	56.30	193	75.98
144	56.69	194	76.38
145	57.09	195	76.77
146	57.48	196	77.17
147	57.87	197	77.56
148	58.27	198	77.95
149	58.66	199	78.35
150	59.06	200	78.74

Conversion of pounds to grams

Ounces	1 lb	2 lb	3 lb	4 lb	5 lb	6 lb	7 lb	8 lb
				Grams				
0	454	907	1361	1814	2268	2722	3175	3629
1	482	936	1389	1843	2296	2750	3204	3657
2	510	964	1418	1871	2325	2778	3232	3686
3	539	992	1446	1899	2353	2807	3260	3714
4	567	1021	1474	1928	2381	2835	3289	3742
5	595	1049	1503	1956	2410	2863	3317	3771
6	624	1077	1531	1985	2438	2892	3345	3799
7	652	1106	1559	2013	2466	2920	3374	3827
8	680	1134	1588	2041	2495	2948	3402	3856
9	709	1162	1616	2070	2523	2977	3430	3884
10	737	1191	1644	2098	2552	3005	3459	3912
11	765	1219	1673	2126	2580	3033	3487	3941
12	794	1247	1701	2155	2608	3062	3515	3969
13	822	1276	1729	2183	2637	3090	3544	3997
14	851	1304	1758	2211	2665	3119	3572	4026
15	879	1332	1786	2240	2693	3147	3600	4054

See *Primary Pediatric Care*, ed 3, p. 1821.

Ways to develop cultural sensitivity

1. Recognize that cultural diversity exists.
2. Demonstrate respect for people as unique individuals, with culture as one factor that contributes to their uniqueness.
3. Respect the unfamiliar.
4. Identify and examine your own cultural beliefs.
5. Recognize that some cultural groups have definitions of health and illness as well as practices that attempt to promote health and cure illness, which may differ from the provider's.
6. Be willing to modify health care delivery in keeping with the patient's cultural background.
7. Do not expect all members of one cultural group to behave in exactly the same way.
8. Appreciate that each person's cultural values are ingrained and therefore very difficult to change.

Modified from Stulc DM: The family as a bearer of culture. In Cookfair JM: *Nursing process and practice in the community,* St Louis, 1990, Mosby.

See *Primary Pediatric Care,* ed 3, p. 128.

Major causes of death by age: birth through 24 years, United States, 1992*

Cause of death	Age (yr)					Total no. of deaths
	<1	1-4	5-14	15-24	0-24	
Accidents (E800-E949)	20.5 [4]	9.3 [1]	9.3 [1]	37.8 [1]	22.1 [1]	20,336
Perinatal conditions (760-779)	389 [1]	0.7	0.1	—	17.4 [2]	15,708
Homicide (E960-978)	8.1	2.8 [5]	1.6 [3]	22.2 [2]	10.2 [3]	9362
Congenital anomalies (740-759)	186.2 [2]	5.5 [2]	1.2 [4]	1.2	10 [4]	9203
Suicide (E950-959)	—	—	0.9	13.0 [3]	5.6 [5]	5007
Neoplasms (140-239)	3.9	3.5 [3]	3.3 [2]	5.3 [4]	4.1	3809
Infections (001-139; 320-322; 466; 480-487; 590)	29.4 [3]	3.0 [4]	1.0 [5]	2.7 [5]	3.3	3000
Cardiovascular (390-398; 402; 404-429)	17.9 [5]	1.8	0.8	2.7 [5]	2.4	2254
Cerebrovascular (430-438)	4.1	0.3	0.2	0.5	0.5	477
Pulmonary (490-496)	1.1	0.4	0.3	0.5	0.4	397
Renal (580-589)	4.7	<0.1	0.1	0.2	0.3	282

Adapted from the National Center for Health Statistics: Advance report of final mortality statistics: 1992, Monthly vital statistics report, vol 43, no 6, suppl, Hyattsville, Md, 1994, Public Health Service.

Figures in parentheses indicate International Classification of Disease, 9th revision, 1975 categories. Figures in brackets indicate ranking (1-5).

*Deaths per 100,000.

Continued.

Major causes of death by age: birth through 24 years, United States, 1992*—cont'd

Cause of death	Age (yr)						Total no. of deaths
	<1	1-4	5-14	15-24	1-14	0-24	
Gastrointestinal (531-33; 540-543; 550-553; 560; 571; 574-575)	2.5	0.1	0.1	0.2	0.1	0.3	278
Anemias (280-285)	1.2	0.4	0.3	0.3	0.3	0.3	302
Diabetes (250)	0.0	0.0	0.2	0.4	0.1	0.2	167
Pregnancy complications (630-676)	0.0	0.0	0.0	0.3	0.0	0.1	111
Nutritional deficiencies (260-269)	0.5	0.0	0.1	0.0	0.0	0.0	40
All other external causes (E980-E999)	1.0	0.2	0.1	0.9	0.1	0.5	461
All other diseases	194.7	8.5	3.3	7.2	4.9	14	12,939
Total (rate)	865.7	43.6	22.5	95.6	28.8	91.3	
Estimated population (thousands)	4000	15,512	36,542	36,147	51,964	92,111	84,133
Number of deaths	34,628	6764	8193	34,548	14,957	84,133	84,133

Adapted from the National Center for Health Statistics: Advance report of final mortality statistics: 1992, Monthly vital statistics report, vol 43, no 6, suppl, Hyattsville, Md, 1994, Public Health Service.

Figures in parentheses indicate International Classification of Disease, 9th revision, 1975 categories. Figures in brackets indicate ranking (1-5).

*Deaths per 100,000.

See *Primary Pediatric Care*, ed 3, p. 19.

Guidelines for newborn urine drug screening

1. The following neonates should have their urine sent for toxicology screens:
   a. Neonates of mothers who have admitted substance abuse
   b. Neonates of mothers who have a past or present history of maternal drug use
   c. Neonates whose mothers exhibit behaviors indicative of substance abuse during labor or delivery, including drug-related or bizarre behavior such as slurred speech, unsteady gait, inappropriate affect, and confusion
   d. Neonates who evidence symptoms of drug intoxication or withdrawal (e.g., sneezing, jitteriness, irritability, high pitch cry, seizure or other neurological symptoms)
2. The following neonates also may have urine sent for toxicology upon assessment and review by a physician:
   a. Neonates of mothers who have had no prenatal care
   b. Neonates not delivered in-hospital.
   c. Cases of abruptio placenta
   d. Cases of congenital syphilis or those whose mother has had a positive syphilis screening test (e.g., VDRL, RPR, FTA)

From the Division of Neonatology, Department of Pediatrics, Albert Einstein College of Medicine/Montefiore Medical Center, Bronx, NY.

See *Primary Pediatric Care,* ed 3, p. 224.

Recommended sizes of endotracheal tubes*

Patient's age	No. (Fr)	Internal diameter (mm)	Length (cm)	Adapter, internal diameter (mm)
Newborn				
<1 kg	11-12	2.5	10	3
>1 kg	13-14	3.0	11	3
1-6 mo	15-16	3.5	11	4
7-12 mo	17-18	4.0	12	4
13-18 mo	19-20	4.5	13	5
19-36 mo	21-22	5.0	14	5
3-4 yr	23-24	5.5	16	6
5 yr	25	6.0	18	6
6-7 yr	26	6.5	18	7
8-9 yr	27-28	7.0	20	7
10-11 yr	29-30	7.5	22	8
12-14 yr	32-34	8.0	24	8

*Tube should be of material labeled "I.T.-Z79" to satisfy standard tissue implant tests.

See *Primary Pediatric Care,* ed 3, p. 1817.

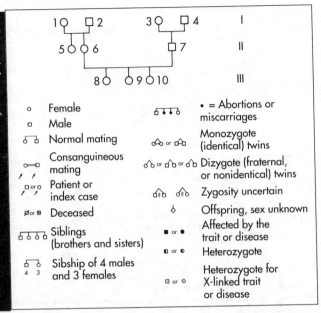

Chart and symbols used to construct a family history, or family
pedigree. The Roman numerals indicate generations.
See *Primary Pediatric Care*, ed 3, p. 48.

Fluoride supplement dosage schedule*

Age	Concentration of fluoride in drinking water (ppm)		
	<0.3	0.3-0.6	>0.6
Birth-6 mo	0	0	0
6 mo-3 yr	0.25	0	0
3-6 yr	0.5	0.25	0
6-16 yr	1	0.5	0

*Dosage regimen accepted by the American Academy of Pediatrics, the American Academy of Pediatric Dentistry (1994), and the American Dental Association (1994).

See *Primary Pediatric Care,* ed 3, p. 263.

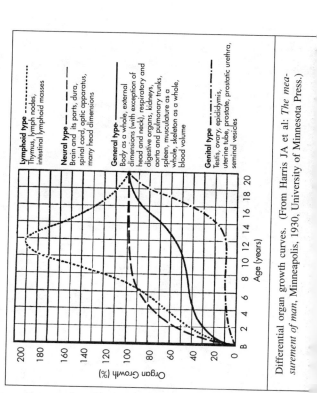

Differential organ growth curves. (From Harris JA et al: *The measurement of man,* Minneapolis, 1930, University of Minnesota Press.)

See *Primary Pediatric Care,* ed 3, p. 58.

Heart rate

Average heart rate for infants and children at rest

Age	Average rate	Two standard deviations
Birth	140	50
First month	130	45
1-6 mo	130	45
6-12 mo	115	40
1-2 yr	110	40
2-4 yr	105	35
6-10 yr	95	30
10-14 yr	85	30
14-18 yr	82	25

From Lowrey GH: *Growth and development of children,* ed 8, Chicago, 1986, Mosby.

See *Primary Pediatric Care,* ed 3, p. 58.

Recommended childhood immunization schedule—United States, January 1996*

Vaccine	Birth	1 mo	2 mo	4 mo	6 mo	12 mo	15 mo	18 mo	4-6 yr	11-12 yr	14-16 yr
Hepatitis B†‡	Hep B-1		Hep B-2		Hep B-3					Hep B‡	
Diphtheria, tetanus, pertussis§			DTP	DTP	DTP	DTP§ (DTaP at 15 + m)			DTP or DTaP	Td	
H. influenzae type b‖			Hib	Hib	Hib‖	Hib‖					
Polio‖			OPV¶	OPV	OPV		OPV		OPV		
Measles, mumps, rubella#						MMR			MMR# or MMR#	MMR#	
Varicella-zoster virus vaccine**							Var			Var**	

From American Academy of Pediatric Committee on Infectious Diseases: *Pediatrics* 97:143, 1996.

*Approved by the Advisory Committee on Immunization Practices (ACIP), the American Academy of Pediatrics (AAP), and the American Academy of Family Physicians (AAFP). Vaccines are listed under the routinely recommended ages. Bars indicate range of acceptable ages for vaccination. Shaded bars indicate catch-up vaccination: at 11-12 years of age, hepatitis B vaccine should be administered to children not previously vaccinated, and varicella-zoster virus vaccine should be administered to children not previously vaccinated who lack a reliable history of chickenpox.

Continued.

†*Infants born to HBsAg-negative mothers* should receive 2.5 µg of Merck vaccine (Recombivax HB) or 10 µg of SmithKline Beecham (SB) vaccine (Engerix-B). The second dose should be administered ≥1 month after the first dose. *Infants born to HBsAg-positive mothers* should receive 0.5 mL hepatitis B immune globulin (HBIG) within 12 hours of birth and either 5 µg of Merck vaccine (Recombivax HB) or 10 µg of SB vaccine (Engerix-B) at a separate site. The second dose is recommended at 1 to 2 months of age and the third dose at 6 months of age. *Infants born to mothers whose HBsAg status is unknown* should receive either 5 µg of Merck vaccine (Recombivax HB) or 10 µg of SB vaccine (Engerix-B) within 12 hours of birth. The second dose of vaccine is recommended at 1 month of age and the third dose at 6 months of age.

‡Adolescents who have not previously received three doses of hepatitis B vaccine should initiate or complete the series at the 11- to 12-year-old visit. The second dose should be administered at least 1 month after the first dose, and the third dose should be administered at least 4 months after the first dose and at least 2 months after the second dose.

§DTaP may be administered at 12 months of age, provided at least 6 months have elapsed since DTP3. DTaP (diphtheria and tetanus toxoids and acellular pertussis vaccine) is licensed for the fourth and/or fifth vaccine dose(s) for children 15 months of age or older and may be preferred for these doses in this age group. Td (tetanus and diphtheria toxoids, adsorbed, for adult use) is recommended at 11 to 12 years of age if at least 5 years have elapsed since the last dose of DTP, DTaP, or DT.

‖Three *H. influenzae* type b (Hib) conjugate vaccines are licensed for use in infants. If PRP-OMP (PedvaxHIB [Merck]) is administered at 2 and 4 months of age, a dose a 6 months is not required. After completing the primary series, any Hib conjugate vaccine may be used as a booster.

¶Oral poliovirus vaccine (OPV) is recommended for routine infant vaccination. Inactivated poliovirus vaccine (IPV) is recommended for persons with a congenital or acquired immune deficiency disease or an altered immune status as a result of disease or immunosuppressive therapy, as well as their household contacts, and is an acceptable alternative for other persons. The primary three-dose series for IPV should be given with a minimum interval of 4 weeks between the first and second doses and 6 months between the second and third doses.

#The second dose of MMR is routinely recommended at 4 to 6 years of age or at 11 to 12 years of age but may be administered at any visit, provided at least 1 month has elapsed since receipt of the first dose.

**Varicella-zoster virus vaccine (Var) can be administered to susceptible children any time after 12 months of age. Unvaccinated children who lack a reliable history of chickenpox should be vaccinated at the 11- to 12-year-old visit.

See *Primary Pediatric Care*, ed 3, p. 184.

Recommended immunization schedule for children not immunized in the first year of life

Recommended time/age	Immunization(s)*†	Comments
		Younger than 7 years
First visit	DTP, Hib, HBV, MMR, OPV	If indicated, tuberculin testing may be done at same visit.
		If child is 5 yr of age or older, Hib is not indicated.
Interval after first visit:		
1 mo	DTP, HBV	OPV may be given if accelerated poliomyelitis vaccination is necessary, such as for travelers to areas where polio is endemic.
2 mo	DTP, Hib, OPV	Second dose of Hib is indicated only in children whose first dose was received when younger than 15 mo.
≥8 mo	DTP or DTaP,‡ HBV, OPV	OPV is not given if the third dose was given earlier.
	DTP or DTaP,‡ OPV	DTP or DTaP is not necessary if the fourth dose was given after the fourth birthday; OPV
4-6 yr (at or before school entry)		is not necessary if the third dose was given after the fourth birthday.
11-12 yr	MMR	At entry to middle school or junior high school.
10 yr later	Td	Repeat every 10 yr throughout life.

Continued.

Recommended immunization schedule for children not immunized in the first year of life—cont'd

Recommended time/age	Immunization(s)*†	Comments
		7 Years and older§‖
First visit	HBV,¶ OPV, MMR, Td	
Interval after first visit:		
2 mo	HBV,¶ OPV, Td	OPV may also be given 1 mo after the first visit if accelerated poliomyelitis vaccination is necessary.
8-14 mo	HBV,¶ OPV, Td	OPV is not given if the third dose was given earlier.
11-12 yr	MMR	At entry to middle school or junior high.
10 yr later	Td	Repeat every 10 yr throughout life.

From Peter G, editor: *1994 Red Book: Report of the Committee on Infectious Diseases,* ed 23, Elk Grove Village, Ill, 1994, American Academy of Pediatrics.

*If all needed vaccines cannot be administered simultaneously, priority should be given to protecting the child against those diseases that pose the greatest immediate risk. In the United States, these diseases for children younger than 2 years usually are measles and *Haemophilus influenzae* type b infection; for children older than 7 years, they are measles, mumps, and rubella (MMR).

†DTP or DTaP, HBV, Hib, MMR, and OPV can be given simultaneously at separate sites if failure of the patient to return for future immunizations is a concern.

‡DTaP is not currently licensed for use in children younger than 15 mo of age and is not recommended for primary immunization (i.e., first three doses) at any age.

Note: For varicella-zoster virus vaccine, see Table 17-1.

§If person is 18 yr or older, routine poliovirus vaccination is not indicated in the United States.

‖Minimal interval between doses of MMR is 1 month.

¶Priority shold be given to hepatitis B immunization of adolescents.

Note: For varicella-zoster virus vaccine, see p. 247.

See *Primary Pediatric Care,* ed 3, p. 185.

Hepatitis B prophylaxis for perinatal and household exposure

1. Infants born to mothers who test positive for hepatitis B antigens have a great probability of being infected (HB_sAg positive, 25% probability; HB_eAg positive, 85% probability). Infection may occur anytime in the first year after birth.
2. Infants infected with HBV have a 90% probability of becoming chronic HBV carriers.
3. Perinatal administration of HBIG is 75% effective in preventing chronic infection.
4. Perinatal administration of HBIG and the HBV vaccine is 90% effective in preventing chronic infection.
5. Both HBIG and the HBV vaccine are recommended.

	Perinatal exposure	**Household contact**
HBIG		
Dose	0.5 ml IM	For infants <12 months of age only
Timing	Within 12 hr of birth	
HBV		
Dose	0.5 ml IM	0.5 ml IM
Timing	Within 2 mo of birth, repeated at 1 mo and 6 mo after the initial dose (may be given at the same time as HBIG and other childhood immunizations)	When contact is identified; repeat after 1 mo and 6 mo

See *Primary Pediatric Care,* ed 3, p. 189.

Conditions warranting administration of influenza vaccine in children

Chronic pulmonary disease (e.g., cystic fibrosis, asthma, severe scoliosis, bronchopulmonary dysplasia, and neuromotor diseases that compromise ventilation)
Heart disease with altered circulatory dynamics
Chronic renal disease with azotemia
Diabetes mellitus and other metabolic diseases
Immunocompromised conditions
Severe chronic anemias

See *Primary Pediatric Care,* ed 3, p. 190.

Guide to tetanus prophylaxis in wound management*

| | Type of wound and type of vaccine given | | |
History of tetanus immunization	Clean minor wound	Moderately tetanus prone	Very tetanus prone
Incomplete or uncertain	Td	Td + TIG-H (250 U)	Td + TIG-H (250-500 U)
Fully immunized but >10 yr since last dose of Td	Td	Td	Td
Fully immunized but 5-10 yr since last dose of Td	None	Td	Td
Fully immunized but <5 yr since last dose of Td	None	None	None

*Schedule recommended by the U.S. Public Health Service's Advisory Committee on Immunization Practices.
Td, Tetanus and diphtheria toxoids (adult type); *TIG-H,* Tetanus immunoglobulin–human, a specific tetanus antitoxin collected from human volunteers.
NOTE: 1. Children under age 7 should be given DTP rather than Td.
    2. A full primary series comprises two doses of tetanus toxoid 2 months apart, plus a booster dose at least 6 months after the second dose.

See *Primary Pediatric Care,* ed 3, p. 186.

Ways to avoid malpractice suits

Standards

· Meet normative standards of health care delivery (i.e., according to expert opinion as found in medical textbooks and articles in scientific journals) and/or empiric standards (i.e., according to local medical practice).

Communication

· Use positive methods in communicating with patients and parents, showing respect, understanding, concern, and compassion.
· Train staff to be sensitive to a patient's needs at all times.
· Train staff to manage patient telephone calls properly and to log all incoming and outgoing telephone calls, including patient problems and instructions given.

Documentation

· Record on the first page of a patient's chart his or her drug allergies and problem list.
· Record for each visit the history, findings on physical examination (including pertinent negative findings), diagnostic tests ordered (including their results), and treatment prescribed in sufficient detail for purposes of recall.
· Record all immunizations given and all screening test results.
· Record all telephone calls during which medical information about the patient was received or advice was given; include date and time.
· Place in the patient's chart discharge summaries of hospitalizations and referral letters to and responses from consultants.

Malpractice avoidance

See *Primary Pediatric Care,* ed 3, p. 9.

Perinatal conditions that increase the risk of neonatal asphyxia

Antepartum conditions

1. Diabetes
2. Toxemia
3. Hypertension
4. Rh sensitization
5. Previous stillbirth or neonatal death
6. Third trimester bleeding
7. Maternal infection
8. Polyhydramnios
9. Oligohydramnios
10. Postterm gestation
11. Multiple gestation
12. Intrauterine growth retardation

Intrapartum conditions

1. Operative delivery
    a. Cesarean section
    b. Midforceps delivery
2. Breech or other abnormal presentation
3. Premature labor
4. Ruptured membranes (>24 hr)
5. Chorioamnionitis
    a. Maternal fever, tachycardia, or both
    b. Ruptured membranes (>24 hr)
    c. Tender uterus
    d. Foul-smelling amniotic fluid
6. Prolonged labor (>24 hr)
7. Fetal distress
    a. Fetal tachycardia (>160 beats/min)
    b. Fetal bradycardia (<120 beats/min)
    c. Persistent late decelerations
    d. Severe variable decelerations without baseline variability
    e. Scalp pH ≤7.25
    f. Meconium-stained amniotic fluid
    g. Cord prolapse
8. General anesthesia
9. Narcotics administered during labor
10. Abruptio placentae
11. Placenta previa

See *Primary Pediatric Care,* ed 3, p. 493.

Equipment required for resuscitation of the newborn

Ventilation

1. Oxygen source—oxygen, warmed and humidified
2. Suction—De Lee suction trap, wall suction with adjustable pressure gauge; suction catheters; sizes 6, 8, 10, 12 Fr
3. Ventilation bag—500 ml self-inflating type with reservoir (capable of delivering 100% O_2) or 500 cc anesthesia type
4. Face masks—infant sizes, premature and term
5. Laryngoscope—blade sizes 0 and 1, spare batteries, and bulbs
6. Endotracheal tubes—sizes 2.5, 3, and 3.5 mm with plastic adapters attached
7. Soft metal stylets for endotracheal tubes
8. Stethoscope
9. Feeding tube—8 Fr tubes to evacuate stomach contents

Temperature control

1. Evaporation—warm towels
2. Conduction—mattress covered with prewarmed towels
3. Convection—air conditioning turned down; delivery room temperature 75° F (23.9° C) minimum
4. Radiation—radiant warmer

Circulation and biochemical resuscitation

1. Umbilical catheterization tray
2. Drugs and volume expanders

Other

50 ml syringe with three-way stopcock and 21-gauge butterfly needle for evacuation of pneumothorax

See *Primary Pediatric Care*, ed 3, p. 493.

Normal values for arterial blood (pH, gases, oxygen saturation, bicarbonate)

Parameter	Unit	Infants and children			Newborn
		Mixed venous	Capillary	Arterial	
pH	units	7.31-7.41	7.35-7.40	7.40-7.45	7.11-7.30
PCO$_2$	torr	35-40	40-45	35-40	27-40
PO$_2$	torr	41-51	45-50	80-100	33-75
SaO$_2$	%	60-80	>70	>90	40-90
HCO$_3^-$	mEq/L	22-25	22-26	22-26	14-22

Modified from Gordon IB: Reference ranges for laboratory tests. In Behrman RE, Vaughan VC, editors: *Nelson's textbook of pediatrics*, ed 12, Philadelphia, 1983, WB Saunders.

HCO$_3^-$, Bicarbonate; *PCO$_2$*, carbon dioxide pressure; *PO$_2$*, oxygen pressure; *SaO$_2$*, saturation.

See *Primary Pediatric Care*, ed 3, p. 1793.

Percentage of body surface area (BSA) in relation to age

Body part	Percent BSA by age				
	Infant	1-4 Years	5-9 Years	10-14 Years	Adult
Parts that change with age					
Head	19	17	13	11	7
Each thigh	5.5	6.5	8	8.5	9.5
Each leg	5	5	5.5	6	7
Parts that do not change with age					
Neck	2				
Anterior trunk	13				
Posterior trunk	13				
Buttocks	5				
Genitalia	1				
Both arms	14				
Both hands	5				
Both feet	7				

See *Primary Pediatric Care,* ed 3, p. 350.

Ranges of body surface area, weight, and vital signs for infants, children, and adults

Age	Body surface area (m²)	Weight (kg)	Pulse*/min	Systolic blood pressure† (mm Hg)	Respiratory rate‡/min
Newborn	0.19	3.5	90-200	60	30-60
1 mo	0.30	4.0	90-180	65	30-60
6 mo	0.38	7.0	90-180	70	24-30
1-2 yr	0.50-0.55	10-12	70-140	72-74	20-24
3-5 yr	0.54-0.68	15-20	60-120	76-80	16-22
6-9 yr	0.68-0.85	20-28	60-120	82-88	14-20
10-12 yr	1.00-1.07	30-38	60-110	90	12-20
12-14 yr	1.07-1.22	38-48	50-100	90	12-20
15-16 yr	1.30-1.60	53-58	50-100	90	12-18
Adult	1.40-1.70	60-70	50-100	90	12-18

Age	mm Hg
0-1 mo	<60
1 mo-1 yr	<70
>1 yr	Formula: 70 + (2 × Age in years)§

Age	Tachypnea rate	Bradypnea rate
<1 yr	>60	<25
1-5 yr	>40	<15
>5 yr	>30	<10

*Pulse range includes sound sleep and vigorous crying.
†Systolic blood pressure less than fifth percentile.
‡Respiratory rate >60 or <10/min is abnormal at any age.
§Formula for 50th percentile systolic BP at 2 to 10 yr is 90 + (2 × Age in years); the diastolic BP is two thirds of the systolic BP.

See *Primary Pediatric Care*, ed 3, p. 1788.

Cerebrospinal fluid analysis: normal values

	Mean	Range	Polymorphonuclear cells
Cell count*			
Preterm newborn	9.0	0-29	57%
Term newborn	8.2	0-32	61%
Child (>1 mo)		0-6	
Glucose			
Preterm newborn	50 mg/dl	24-63 mg/dl	
Term newborn	52 mg/dl	34-119 mg/dl	
Child		40-80 mg/dl	
Pressure, opening			
Newborn	<110 mm H_2O		
Child	<200 mm H_2O		
Protein			
Preterm newborn	115 mg/dl	65-150 mg/dl	
Term newborn	90 mg/dl	20-170 mg/dl	
Child		5-40 mg/dl	
Volume			
Child	60-100 ml		
Adult	100-160 ml		

Modified from Klein JO, Feigin RD, McCracken GH: *Pediatrics* 78(suppl):959, 1986; Portnoy JM, Olson LC: *Pediatrics* 75:484, 1985; Sarff LD, Platt LH, McCracken GH: *J Pediatr* 88:473, 1976.

*Traumatic lumbar punctures (>1000 red blood cells/mm^3) are uninterpretable because correction formulas may underestimate the true white blood cell count.

See *Primary Pediatric Care*, ed 3, p. 1821.

Normal newborn clinical chemistry values

Determination*	Cord sample†	Capillary samples†			
		1-12 hr	12-24 hr	24-48 hr	48-72 hr
Sodium (mmol/L)	147 (126-166)	143 (124-156)	145 (132-159)	148 (134-160)	149 (139-162)
Potassium (mmol/L)	7.8 (5.6-12)	6.4 (5.3-7.3)	6.3 (5.3-8.9)	6.0 (5.2-7.3)	5.9 (5.0-7.7)
Chloride (mmol/L)	103 (98-110)	100.7 (90-111)	103 (87-114)	102 (92-114)	103 (93-112)
Calcium (mg/dl)	9.3 (8.2-11.1)	8.4 (7.3-9.2)	7.8 (6.9-9.4)	8.0 (6.1-9.9)	7.9 (5.9-9.7)
Phosphorus (mg/dl)	5.6 (3.7-8.1)	6.1 (3.5-8.6)	5.7 (2.9-8.1)	5.9 (3.0-8.7)	5.8 (2.8-7.6)
Blood urea (mg/dl)	29 (21-40)	27 (8-34)	33 (9-63)	32 (13-77)	31 (13-68)
Total protein (g/dl)	6.1 (4.8-7.3)	6.6 (5.6-8.5)	6.6 (5.8-8.2)	6.9 (5.9-8.2)	7.2 (6.0-8.5)
Glucose (mg/dl)	73 (45-96)	63 (40-97)	63 (42-104)	56 (30-91)	59 (40-90)
Lactic acid (mg/dl)	19.5 (11-30)	14.6 (11-24)	14 (10-23)	14.3 (9-22)	13.5 (7-21)
Lactate (mmol/L)‡	2.0-3.0	2.0			

Modified from Avery GB: *Neonatology, pathophysiology and management in the newborn*, ed 3, Philadelphia, 1987, JB Lippincott.
*Acharya PT, Payne WW: *Arch Dis Child* 40:430, 1965.
†Numbers in parentheses indicate a normal range.
‡Daniel SS, Adamsons K Jr, James LS: *Pediatrics* 37:942, 1966.

See *Primary Pediatric Care*, ed 3, p. 1821.

Normal clinical chemistry values

Determination	Standard units	Factor	SI units
Alanine aminotransferase (ALT or SGPT)			
Infant	5-54 U/L	NA	NA
Child	3-37 U/L	NA	NA
Adult	8-45 U/L	NA	NA
Alkaline phosphatase			
Newborn	35-213 U/L	1.00	35-213 U/L
Child	71-142 U/L	1.00	71-142 U/L
Adolescent	106-213 U/L	1.00	106-213 U/L
Adult	32-92 U/L	1.00	32-92 U/L
Aldolase			
Newborn	5.2-32.8 U/L	1.00	5.2-32.8 U/L
Child	2.6-16.4 U/L	1.00	2.6-16.4 U/L
Adult	1.3-8.2 U/L	1.00	1.3-8.2 U/L
Ammonia	15-49 µg/dl	0.7333	11-35 µmol/L
Amylase			
Serum	60-160 U/dl	NA*	NA
Urine	17-200 U/dl	NA	NA
Aspartate aminotransferase (AST or SGOT)			
Newborn	25-75 U/L	NA	NA
Infant	15-60 U/L	NA	NA
Child	20-50 U/L	NA	NA
Adult	8-40 U/L	NA	NA

Continued.

Normal clinical chemistry values—cont'd

Determination	Standard units	Factor	SI units
Bicarbonate	18-25 mEq/L	1.00	8-25 mmol/L
Bilirubin (>1 mo)			
Total	<0.2-1.0 mg/dl	17.10	<3.4 μmol/L
Direct	<0.2 mg/dl	17.10	<3.4-17.1 μmol/L
Calcium			
Total	8.8-10.8 mg/dl	0.2495	2.20-2.70 mmol/L
Ionized	4.48-4.92 mg/dl	0.2495	1.12-1.23 mmol/L
Carotene			
Infant	20-70 μg/dl	0.0186	0.37-1.30 μmol/L
Adult	40-130 μg/dl	0.0186	0.74-2.42 μmol/L
Child	60-200 μg/dl	0.0186	1.12-3.72 μmol/L
Chloride	98-106 mEq/L	1.00	98-106 mmol/L
Cholesterol, fasting			
Newborn	53-135 mg/dl	0.0259	1.37-3.50 mmol/L
Infant	70-175 mg/dl	0.0259	1.81-4.53 mmol/L
Child	120-200 mg/dl	0.0259	3.11-5.18 mmol/L
Adolescent	120-210 mg/dl	0.0259	3.11-5.44 mmol/L
Adult	140-250 mg/dl	0.0259	3.63-6.48 mmol/L
Copper			
Infant	20-70 μg/dl	0.1574	3.14-10.99 μmol/L
Child	90-190 μg/dl	0.1574	14.13-29.83 μmol/L
Adolescent	80-160 μg/dl	0.1574	12.56-25.12 μmol/L
Adult	70-155 μg/dl	0.1574	10.99-24.34 μmol/L

Creatinine			
Newborn	0.8-1.4 mg/dl	88.4	70.7-123.8 µmol/L
Infant	0.7-1.7 mg/dl	88.4	61.9-150.3 µmol/L
Adult	0.6-1.5 mg/dl	88.4	53.133 µmol/L
Creatinine kinase			
Female	10-55 U/L	1.00	10-55 U/L
Male	12-80 U/L	1.00	12-80 U/L
Glucose	55-100 mg/dl	0.05551	3.055-5.55 mmol/L
Haptoglobin	40-336 mg/dl	0.01	0.4-3.36 g/L
Iron, serum			
Newborn	100-250 µg/dl	0.1791	17.90-44.75 µmol/L
Infant	40-100 µg/dl	0.1791	7.16-17.90 µmol/L
Child	50-120 µg/dl	0.1791	8.95-21.48 µmol/L
Adult	40-160 µg/dl	0.1791	7.16-28.64 µmol/L
Iron-binding capacity, total (TIBC)			
Infant	100-400 µg/dl	0.1791	17.90-71.60 µmol/L
Child	250-400 µg/dl	0.1791	44.75-71.60 µmol/L
Adult	250-400 µg/dl	0.1791	44.75-71.60 µmol/L
Lactate	0.6-1.8 mEq/L	1.00	0.6-1.8 mmol/L
Lactic dehydrogenase			
Newborn	160-450 U/L	NA	NA
Infant	100-250 U/L	NA	NA
Child	60-170 U/L	NA	NA
Adult	45-90 U/L	NA	NA
Lead (child)	<10 µg/dl	0.0483	<0.48 µmol/L
Lipids			
Phospholipids	180-295 mg/dl	0.01	1.8-2.95 g/L
Triglycerides	40-150 mg/dl	0.01	0.4-1.5 g/L

Continued.

Normal clinical chemistry values—cont'd

Determination	Standard units	Factor	SI units
Lipoprotein, HDL	150-330 mg/dl	0.01	1.5-3.3 g/L
Lipoprotein, LDL	28%-53% total		
Magnesium			
Newborn	1.0-1.8 mEq/L	0.5	0.5-0.9 mmol/L
Child	1.5-2.0 mEq/L	0.5	0.8-1.0 mmol/L
Osmolarity	275-295 mOsm/kg	1.00	275-295 mmol/kg
pH (arterial)	7.35-7.45	1.00	7.35-7.45
Proteins (NOTE: Globulin = Total protein − Albumin)			
Albumin/total protein			
Newborn	2.4-4.8/4.6-7.0 g/dl	10.0	24-48/46-70 g/L
Infant	3.0-4.5/5.1-7.3 g/dl	10.0	30-45/51-73 g/L
Child	3.8-5.6/6.0-8.0 g/dl	10.0	38-56/60-80 g/L
Adult	3.5-5.5/6.4-8.3 g/dl	10.0	35-55/64-83 g/L
Sodium	136-145 mEq/L	1.00	136-145 mmol/L
Urea nitrogen			
Newborn	4-12 mg/dl	0.3569	1.4-4.3 mmol/L
Child/adult	5-18 mg/dl	0.3569	1.8-6.4 mmol/L
Uric acid	3.0-7.0 mg/dl	0.0595	0.18-0.42 mmol/L
Vitamin A	30-80 µg/dl	0.0349	1.05-2.79 µmol/L
Vitamin E (tocopherol)	0.5-2.0 mg/dl	23.22	11.6-46.4 µmol/L

*NA, Not available or not applicable.

See *Primary Pediatric Care*, ed 3, p. 1821.

Normal hematological values

Age	Hemoglobin (grams %): mean (−2 SD)	Hematocrit (%) mean (−2 SD)	Mean cell volume (fluid) mean (−2 SD)	Mean corpuscular hemoglobin concentration (grams/%RBC) mean (−2 SD)	Reticulocytes (%)	WBC/mm³ × 100 mean (−2 SD)	Platelets (10³ mm³) mean (±2 SD)
26-30 wk gestation*	13.4 (11)	41.5 (34.9)	118.2 (106.7)	37.9 (30.6)	—	4.4 (2.7)	254
28 wk	14.5	45	120	31	(5-10)	—	(180-327)
32 wk	15.0	47	118	32	(3-10)	—	275
Term† (cord)	16.5 (13.5)	51 (42)	108 (98)	33 (30)	(3-7)	18.1 (9-30)‡	290
1-3 days	18.5 (14.5)	56 (45)	108 (95)	33 (29)	(1.8-4.6)	18.9 (9.4-34)	290
2 wk	16.6 (13.4)	53 (41)	105 (88)	31.4 (28.1)		11.4 (5-20)	192
1 mo	13.9 (10.7)	44 (33)	101 (91)	31.8 (28.1)	(0.1-1.7)	10.8 (4-19.5)	252
2 mo	11.2 (9.4)	35 (28)	95 (84)	31.8 (28.3)			
6 mo	12.6 (11.1)	36 (31)	76 (68)	35 (32.7)	(0.7-2.3)	11.9 (6-17.5)	(150-350)
6 mo-2 yr	12 (10.5)	36 (33)	78 (70)	33 (30)		10.6 (6-17)	(150-350)
2-6 yr	12.5 (11.5)	37 (34)	81 (75)	34 (31)	(0.5-1.0)	8.5 (5-15.5)	(150-350)
6-12 yr	13.5 (11.5)	40 (35)	86 (77)	34 (31)	(0.5-1.0)	8.1 (4.5-13.5)	(150-350)
12-18 yr							
Male	14.5 (13)	43 (36)	88 (78)	34 (31)	(0.5-1.0)	7.8 (4.5-13.5)	(150-350)
Female	14 (12)	41 (37)	90 (78)	34 (31)	(0.5-1.0)	7.8 (4.5-13.5)	(150-350)
Adult							
Male	15.5 (13.5)	47 (41)	90 (80)	34 (31)	(0.8-2.5)	7.4 (4.5-11)	(150-350)
Female	14 (12)	41 (36)	90 (80)	34 (31)	(0.8-4.1)	7.4 (4.5-11)	(150-350)

Modified from Johnson KB, editor: *The Harriet Lane handbook*, ed 13, Chicago, 1993, Mosby.

*Values are from fetal samplings.

†Under 1 mo of age, capillary hemoglobin exceeds venous hemoglobin: age 1 hr—by 3.6 g; age 5 days—by 2.2 g; age 3 wk—by 1.1 g.

See *Primary Pediatric Care*, ed. 3, p. 1821.

Normal hematological values during first 2 weeks of life in term infant

	Cord blood	Day 1	Day 3	Day 7	Day 14
Hemoglobin (g/dl)	16.8	18.4	17.8	17.0	16.8
Hematocrit (%)	53.0	58.0	55.0	54.0	52.0
Red cells (mm^3 × 10^6)	5.25	5.8	5.6	5.2	5.1
MCV (fL)	107.0	108.0	99.0	98.0	96.0
MCH (pg/cell)	34.0	35.0	33.0	32.5	31.5
MCHC (g/dl RBCs)	31.7	32.5	33.0	33.0	33.0
Reticulocytes (%)	3-7	3-7	1-3	0-1	0-1
Nucleated RBC/(mm^3)	500	200	0-5	0	0
Platelets (1000/mm^3)	290	192	213	248	252

From Nathan DG, Oski F: *Hematology of infancy and childhood*, ed 3, Philadelphia, 1987, WB Saunders.
MCV, mean corpuscular volume; *MCH*, mean corpuscular hemoglobin; *MCHC*, mean corpuscular hemoglobin concentration; *RBC*, red blood cells.

See *Primary Pediatric Care*, ed 3, p. 873.

Average weight by age

Age	Weight (kg) Girl	Weight (kg) Boy	Convenient weight to remember (kg)
Newborn	3.4	3.2	3
3 mo	6.0	5.9	6
6 mo	8.5	7.7	
9 mo	9.6	9.0	9
1 yr	10.8	10.0	10
2 yr	13.3	12.5	
3 yr	15.2	14.8	15
4 yr	17.3	16.9	
5 yr	19.5	19.2	20
8 yr	29.4	29.9	30
10 yr	34.9	35.5	35
15 yr	60.1	57.5	60

See *Primary Pediatric Care,* ed 3, p. 341.

Obstructive sleep apnea score

OSA Score = $1.42D + 1.41A + 0.71S - 3.83$

D = Difficulty of breathing during sleep (0 = never, 1 = occasionally, 2 = frequently, and 3 = always)

A = Apnea observed during sleep (0 = No and 1 = yes)

S = Snoring (0 = never, 1 = occasionally, 2 = frequently, and 3 = always)

Scores of >3.5 are highly predictive of the need for T&A

Scores of <−1 rule out OSA

Scores of −1 to 3.4 require polysomography to determine whether OSA requiring T&A exists

See *Primary Pediatric Care,* ed 3, p. 1626.

First aid for snakebites

1. Observe the approximate size and characteristics of the snake if this can be done without danger of remaining within the snake's striking range.
2. Move the patient as little as possible.
3. Mark the victim's skin with a pen denoting the area of swelling and the time. Repeat this every 15 minutes.
4. Remove all rings from the victim's fingers.
5. Immobilize the affected limb by splinting as if for a fracture and keep the limb below the level of the heart.
6. Regardless of early symptoms, transport the victim to the nearest medical facility at a safe speed.
7. Avoid the use of ice (tissue damage), aspirin (anticoagulation), alcohol or sedative drugs (vasodilation), or stimulants such as caffeine (acceleration of venom absorption).
8. As soon as possible start basic life support, including volume expansion and Trendelenburg position for hypotensive patients.

See *Primary Pediatric Care,* ed 3, p. 1696.

Criteria for referral of the child who stutters

	Normal disfluencies Age of onset: 1½ to 7 years of age	Mild stuttering Age of onset: 1½ to 7 years of age	Severe stuttering Age of onset: 1½ to 7 years of age
Speech behaviors you may see or hear	Occasional (not more than once in every 10 sentences), brief (typical ½ second or shorter) repetitions of sounds, syllables, or short words (e.g., "li-li-like this")	Frequent (3% or more of speech), long (½ to 1 second) repetitions of sounds, syllables, or short words, (e.g., "li-li-li-like this"); occasional prolongations of sounds	Very frequent (10% or more of speech) and often very long (1 second or longer) repetitions of sounds, syllables, or short words; frequent sound prolongations and blockages
Other behaviors you may see or hear	Occasional pauses, hesitations in speech, or fillers such as "uh," "er," or "um"; changing of words or thoughts	Repetitions and prolongations begin to be associated with eyelid closing and blinking, looking to the side, and some physical tension in and around the lips	Similar to mild stutterers only more frequent and noticeable; some rise in pitch of voice during stuttering; extra sounds or words used as "starters"
When problem is most noticeable	Come and go when child is tired, excited, talking about complex/new topics, asking or answering questions, or talking to unresponsive listeners	Come and go in similar situations but more often present than absent	Tends to be present in most speaking; far more consistent and nonfluctuating
Child reaction	None apparent	Some show little concern, some will be frustrated and embarrassed	Most are embarrassed and some also fear speaking
Parent reaction	None to a great deal	Most concerned, but concern may be minimal	All have some degree of concern
Referral decision	Refer only if parents moderately to overly concerned	Refer if continues for 6 to 8 weeks or if parental concern justifies it	Refer as soon as possible

Adapted for use by permission of the Stuttering Foundation of America, Memphis, Tenn.

See *Primary Pediatric Care*, ed 3, p. 755.

Stuttering child, referral criteria

Synovial fluid analysis

	Cells per microliter (µl)	Polymorphonuclear leukocytes (PMNL)	Glucose (mg/dl)	Mucin clot	Protein (mg/dl)
Normal	50-200	<5%	>80	Good	1.8
Inflammatory*					
Bacterial	>10,000	>90%	<50	Poor	>4
Nonseptic	<10,000	<90%	50-80	Poor	2-4

Modified from Rudy P, DuPont HL: Infectious arthritis. In Pickering LK, DuPont HL, editors: *Infectious diseases of children and adults,* Menlo Park, Calif, 1986, Addison-Wesley.
*Fluid should be evaluated for the presence of urate crystals that occur in gout and pseudogout.

See *Primary Pediatric Care,* ed 3, p. 1821.

Celsius-Fahrenheit temperature equivalents

Celsius*	Fahrenheit†	Celsius*	Fahrenheit†
34.0	93.2	38.6	101.4
34.2	93.6	38.8	101.8
34.4	93.9	39.0	102.2
34.6	94.3	39.2	102.5
34.8	94.6	39.4	102.9
35.0	95.0	39.6	103.2
35.2	95.4	39.8	103.6
35.4	95.7	40.0	104.0
35.6	96.1	40.2	104.3
35.8	96.4	40.4	104.7
36.0	96.8	40.6	105.1
36.2	97.1	40.8	105.4
36.4	97.5	41.0	105.8
36.6	97.8	41.2	106.1
36.8	98.2	41.4	106.5
37.0	98.6	41.6	106.8
37.2	98.9	41.8	107.2
37.4	99.3	42.0	107.6
37.6	99.6	42.2	108.0
37.8	100.0	42.4	108.3
38.0	100.4	42.6	108.7
38.2	100.7	42.8	109.0
38.4	101.1	43.0	109.4

*To convert Celsius to Fahrenheit: 9/5 × (Temperature) + 32).
†To convert Fahrenheit to Celsius: 5/9 × (Temperature) − 32).

See *Primary Pediatric Care*, ed 3, p. 1821.

Indications advanced for tonsillectomy, adenoidectomy, or both

Absolute indications

Alveolar hypoventilation (obstructive sleep apnea) or cor pulmonale, secondary to airway obstruction

Dysphagia

Malignancy (radiotherapy alone preferred in most cases)

Uncontrollable hemorrhage from tonsillar blood vessels

Nasal obstruction causing discomfort in breathing and severe distortion of speech

Controversial indications

Recurrent peritonsillar abscess

Chronic cervical lymphadenitis

Hyponasality, "hot potato" voice, or both

Chronic or recurrent tonsillitis

Chronic or recurrent otitis media

Sensorineural or conductive hearing loss

Chronic mastoiditis

Cholesteatoma

Chronic sinusitis or nasopharyngitis

Diphtheria or streptococcal carrier state

Chronic bronchitis or pneumonia

Mouth breathing, snoring, or both (without obstructive sleep apnea)

Rheumatic fever, when compliance with antistreptococcal prophylaxis cannot be assured

Parental anxiety

Frequent colds with loss of time from school

Adenoidal facies

Allergic respiratory diseases

Chronic cough

Failure to thrive

Poor appetite

Focus of infection

Halitosis

Scarred or cryptic tonsils

Routine procedure

See *Primary Pediatric Care*, ed 3, p. 1626.

Children at high risk for tuberculosis in the United States

Children who have had contact with adults who are or were:
Foreign-born persons from countries that have a high prevalence of the disease
Residents of correctional institutions
Residents of long-term care facilities
Homeless
Users of intravenous and other street drugs
Poor or medically indigent, especially urban residents
Infected with HIV
From families that have a history of tuberculosis

See *Primary Pediatric Care,* ed 3, p. 1631.

Urinary tract infections: factors that can cause low colony counts in spite of significant infection

High-volume urine flow
Low urine pH (<5.0) and specific gravity (<1.003)
Recent antimicrobial therapy
Fastidious organisms
Use of inappropriate culture techniques
Bacteriostatic agents in the urine
Complete obstruction of a ureter
Chronic or indolent infection

See *Primary Pediatric Care,* ed 3, p. 1641.

Index